WHAT YOU MUST KNOW ABOUT

DIALYSIS

THE SECRETS TO SURVIVING AND THRIVING ON DIALYSIS

RICH SNYDER, DO

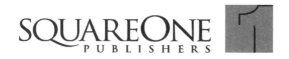

SQUAREONE
PUBLISHERS

The information and advice contained in this book are based upon the research and the personal and professional experiences of the author. They are not intended as a substitute for consulting with a healthcare professional. The publisher and author are not responsible for any adverse effects or consequences resulting from the use of any of the suggestions or procedures discussed in this book. All matters pertaining to your physical health should be supervised by a healthcare professional. It is a sign of wisdom, not cowardice, to seek a second or third opinion.

COVER DESIGNER: Jeannie Tudor
COVER PHOTO: Getty Images, Inc.
INTERIOR ILLUSTRATIONS ON PAGES 21, 37, 39, 40, AND 42: Cathy Morrison
TYPESETTERS: Gary A. Rosenberg & Terry E. Wiscovitch
IN-HOUSE EDITOR: Joanne Abrams

Square One Publishers
115 Herricks Road
Garden City Park, NY 11040
(516) 535-2010 • (877) 900-BOOK
www.squareonepublishers.com

Library of Congress Cataloging-in-Publication Data
Snyder, Rich.
  What you must know about dialysis : the secrets to surviving and thriving on dialysis / Rich Snyder.
      p. cm.
  Includes bibliographical references and index.
  ISBN 978-0-7570-0349-3 (pbk.)
  1. Hemodialysis—Patients. 2. Hemodialysis—Popular works. I. Title. II. Title: Dialysis.
  RC901.7.H45S64 2013
  617.4'61059—dc23
                              2012028692

Printed in the United States of America

10   9   8   7   6   5   4   3   2   1

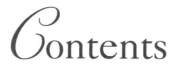

Contents

I dedicate this book to Patty Paul, RN.
The epitome of what a dialysis nurse should be,
she brought out the best in all who came in contact with her.
In addition to being a great nurse,
she was my friend, and will never be forgotten.

I also dedicate this book to my mother, Nancy Snyder, RN.
Without her, this book would not have been possible.

Finally, I dedicate this book to dialysis nurses
and dialysis technicians everywhere. You give your time,
your hearts, and your souls each and every day.
From the bottom of my heart, thank you.

Acknowledgments

I would like to thank everyone I work with at LVNA. You keep each day interesting; there is never a dull moment.

I would also like to acknowledge the dialysis nurses everywhere. I thank you for your tireless efforts to improve the lives of those around you. You are greatly appreciated.

To those on dialysis everywhere, I thank you for allowing me into your lives. I applaud your courage, your fortitude, and your toughness.

To Rudy Shur and Anthony Pomes at Square One Publishers, thank you for your support and encouragement and for putting up with my sometimes endless emails. To Joanne Abrams, thank you for your help and infinite patience.

Finally, I am grateful for the information that has been provided by Dr. Natarajan Ranganathan, Dr. Ira Taffner, John Kirton, Yvonne Anderson, and Bruno Hoffman.

A NOTE ON GENDER

To avoid long and awkward phrasing within sentences, it is our publishing style to alternate the use of male and female pronouns according to the chapter. This means that when referring to a "third-person" patient or caregiver, odd-numbered chapters will use male pronouns, and even numbered chapters will use female pronouns.

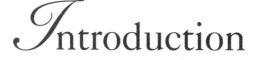

Introduction

Dialysis—the use of an artificial filter to clean and purify the blood—can be a lifesaving technique for the individual whose kidneys are unable to remove toxic waste and excess water from the blood. But if you don't know much about this treatment, dialysis can also seem more than a little scary and overwhelming. What exactly happens during dialysis? How are you likely to feel during and after treatment? And how will these treatments affect your health and your everyday life?

This book was designed to take the fear and uncertainty out of dialysis by explaining—clearly and simply—all the fundamentals of this medical procedure. But *What You Must Know About Dialysis* is far more than a guide to treatments. I firmly believe that to have the best possible experience and enjoy the best health, you have to take an active role in your own care. That's why, throughout these pages, I emphasize the choices you can make to improve your treatments, your overall well-being, and your day-to-day life. I look not only at your options regarding the dialysis process, but also at how you can enhance your health through good dietary choices, nutritional supplements, and exercise. My approach is holistic, which means that in addition to considering physical health, I also examine emotional, spiritual, and social well-being, all of which can have a profound impact on your physical condition.

What You Must Know About Dialysis is divided into two Parts. Part One, entitled "Understanding the Fundamentals of Dialysis," was written to answer all of your questions about dialysis and associated treatments and therapies. You will start by learning about the basic functions performed by healthy kidneys, and then explore the conditions under which dialysis becomes necessary. Other chapters explain your dialysis options, including home and in-center treatments; tell you everything you need to know about the different types of dialysis access, including how you can best care for and protect this "lifeline"; detail your monthly blood work; and introduce you to the medications your physician may prescribe to address dialysis-related issues such as anemia or weak bones. Throughout, I strive to give you the facts you need to be an active participant in your treatments.

Entitled "Taking Action," Part Two provides a wealth of information on the many ways in which you can improve your dialysis sessions and your overall health. This section of the book begins by focusing on two issues that are of great importance to every dialysis patient—fluid balance and blood pressure. By taking steps to control these factors, you will find that you feel better both during and between treatments. Other topics include how you can best take those medications that are not related to dialysis; how you and your doctor can choose nutritional supplements that can enhance your energy, combat inflammation, strengthen your bones, and support heart function; and how you can put together a healthy dialysis diet. In Part Two, you will also learn how you can improve your health by strengthening your body, mind, and spirit. Finally, you will discover the fundamentals of kidney transplants, the gold standard of kidney treatments, and you will explore the top ten "secrets" to improving your dialysis sessions.

While I have tried to make every discussion in this book as clear and easy-to-follow as possible, dialysis is a complicated subject, as is the overall topic of health. That's why, on page 169, I've included a Glossary that will help you understand not only the terminology found in this book, but also the terms that may be used by the professionals on your healthcare team. It's vital that you communicate with your team—about how you're feeling, about how you're responding to treatments, and about ways in which you can improve your care. This Glossary will help you out when the discussions get a bit technical. On page 177, a Resources section will let you know about websites and organizations that can provide further information about topics of interest, and will steer you to companies that offer a range of health-enhancing products.

I cannot overstate the fact that you are a vital member of your own health team, and that you will reap the most benefits from your treatments if you participate in your own care. With the help of this book, I promise that you will learn the secrets to not just surviving but truly thriving on dialysis, physically, emotionally, and spiritually. Let's get started!

PART ONE

Understanding the Fundamentals of Dialysis

If you've recently been told that you need dialysis, you probably have a lot of questions. Why exactly do you require dialysis? What does dialysis do? How does it work? Are there different types of dialysis? Part One was written to answer these questions—and many more—by clearly explaining the fundamentals of dialysis.

Chapter 1 begins at the beginning by telling you about the basic functions performed by healthy kidneys. This information is essential to an understanding of dialysis, since the therapy is designed to do two of the most important jobs of the kidneys—filter toxins out of the bloodstream and control the buildup of excess fluids. Chapter 1 also looks at the many factors that nephrologists (kidney doctors) consider before putting someone on dialysis. By the time you're finished with this chapter, you will have a better understanding of why your physician has recommended this treatment.

Chapter 2 answers the important question, "What are my dialysis options?" The chapter covers the two main types of dialysis—hemodialysis and peritoneal dialysis—briefly describing what each one involves. Within hemodialysis, there are three different plans of treatment—in-center, nocturnal, and home—and you'll learn about them, as well. To help you choose the best type of dialysis for both your health and your lifestyle, I've included a section that evaluates some important factors, such as how each option is likely to affect your diet, your medication regimen, and family and social activities. There is even a discussion of switching dialysis modalities, so this chapter has value whether you're contemplating treatment for the first time or are already receiving dialysis.

Chapter 3 explains the importance of the dialysis access—the specially created entryway into your bloodstream that allows treatments to take place. As you will learn, your dialysis access is your lifeline, and it merits serious consideration. This chapter talks about the various options from which your medical team can choose, explains how each is created, and guides you in taking care of your access to keep it in the best shape possible.

In Chapter 4, you'll read about the blood work that will be performed every month that you're on dialysis. You'll learn why each of the tests is done—to determine the status of your bones, your blood, or another aspect of your health—and what the results mean about the success of your treatments. As you may already know, your dialysis team will give you a monthly report of your blood work and encourage you to become familiar with it. This chapter not only explains why these reports are so important, but also enables you to turn them into a valuable picture of your physical well-being.

Chapter 5, the final portion of Part One, is the perfect complement to Chapter 4 because while Chapter 4 explores issues such as bone and blood health, Chapter 5 discusses the medications that your doctor may prescribe to deal with these issues. You'll discover what each medication is, what it does, and how it should be taken for the best results possible. Finally, you'll find some proven strategies for working your medication regimen into your daily life.

If you are learning about dialysis for the first time—and even if you've already begun treatment—the sheer volume of "things you need to know" can be overwhelming. Yes, there is a lot to know about dialysis, but learning it doesn't have to be an overwhelming or difficult process. The following pages will provide you with the fundamental information you need to understand your medical condition, make the best decisions regarding your healthcare, and become an active participant in your treatments.

1

*W*hen Is Dialysis Needed?

People discover that they need kidney dialysis under a variety of circumstances. Perhaps you have been treated for chronic kidney disease (CKD) for years, and now, your kidney function has decreased to a point where you need the help of an artificial organ—in other words, dialysis. Or perhaps during testing and treatment for another condition, such as congestive heart failure, your doctor discovered that that your kidneys are not doing their job. Whatever the circumstance, you now know that you will require dialysis in the near future or, perhaps, right away. And you probably have a lot of questions.

This chapter will start the process of answering your questions by explaining why dialysis is needed. It first provides information on healthy kidneys—where they're found and what they do. This is important, because without an understanding of healthy kidneys, it's difficult to understand what occurs when the kidneys fail to work properly. You'll then learn about the stages of kidney disease and the most important indications for dialysis.

WHERE ARE THE KIDNEYS LOCATED?

The kidneys are located behind the belly, one on either side of the spinal column. They are found underneath the ribs right where your mid-back (thoracic spine) meets your lower back (lumbar spine). The right kidney sits a little lower than the left. In an average-sized person, the kidneys are approximately four inches in length, but their size can vary depending on a person's body size and degree and duration of kidney disease.

Each kidney is connected to a small, tube-like structure called a *ureter (your-i-ter)* that serves as a bridge between the kidney and bladder. Urine is formed in the kidneys and then flows through the ureters into the bladder, which is the temporary holding tank. When the bladder is full, the urine exits the body through another tube-like structure called the *urethra (your-wreath-ra)*. Together, the kidneys, ureters, bladder, and urethra make up the body's urinary tract, shown in Figure 1.1.

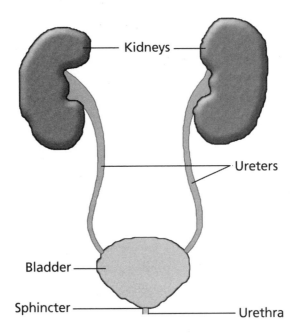

Figure 1.1. Front View of the Urinary Tract.
Each kidney is connected to a tube called a ureter, which leads to the bladder. Urine formed in the kidneys flows through the ureters to the bladder, and eventually leaves the body through the urethra.

WHAT DO THE KIDNEYS DO?

Although the kidneys are best known for their important function of filtering the blood, they actually perform several other vital functions, as well. Below, you'll learn about the chief roles these organs play in the body.

Filtering the Blood

As the body's filters, the kidneys clean and purify the blood by eliminating toxins as waste. Think of a pool pump filter. The pool water flows into the pump and through the filter, where the waste products are removed. The filtered water is then pumped back into the pool. In the body, blood flows into the kidneys, where the toxins are removed. Unlike the pool analogy, however, after the blood is filtered, the byproduct—urine—is excreted.

Your kidneys clean your blood—twenty-four hours a day, seven days a week—via millions of small blood filters called *glomeruli (glo-mare-ewl-eye)*. When we discuss kidney function, the focus is on how well the glomeruli, which are actually networks of tiny blood vessels, are collectively doing their job. In other words, in evaluating kidney function, your doctor is looking for the answer to one question: "How well are the kidneys functioning as filters?"

Additionally, the kidneys have a kind of "sixth sense," in that as they filter the blood, they instinctively know when the body is out of balance. When it is, the kidneys correct it. For example, when someone eats too much high-sodium food, normally functioning kidneys remove the excess sodium the body doesn't need, keeping the body in balance. In much the same way, the kidneys are programmed to keep blood levels of the minerals potassium, calcium, and magnesium within a normal range. These basic, life-sustaining components are called *electrolytes (elek-tro-lites)*. Regulation of their levels is important to maintaining total body balance.

Maintaining Acid-Base Balance

In addition to regulating levels of the electrolytes discussed above, the kidneys help control an important electrolyte called *bicarbonate (bye-carb-o-net)*, which is your body's equivalent of baking soda—a very strong base. Going back to the pool analogy, every pool owner learns how to maintain the water's proper acid-base level, or pH. In a similar way, the kidneys' role is to maintain the body's acid-base balance.

Malfunctioning kidneys can cause bicarbonate levels to fall. When this happens, the acid level in the blood can rise, and over a period of time, the acid buildup can be toxic to the body.

Regulating Blood Pressure

The kidneys also help regulate blood pressure. In addition to eliminating excess sodium from the body, which helps maintain normal blood pressure, they are responsible for the production of the blood pressure hormones called *renin (wren-in)*, and *angiotensin (angie-o-tense-in)*. The kidneys make these two hormones when blood pressure is low. Moreover, the *adrenal (a-dree-null) gland*, which sits on top of the kidneys, makes a third hormone called *aldosterone (al-dost-tair-own)*. The job of these three hormones is to raise blood pressure.

Unfortunately, these hormones—referred to as the *renin-angiotensin-aldosterone (RAA)* system—can also adversely affect the kidneys. They can elicit inflammatory changes in people with kidney disease, and they can contribute to the worsening of kidney function for people with high blood pressure, diabetes, and many other conditions that can cause kidney disease.

Maintaining Blood and Bone Health

The kidneys are major players in maintaining both blood and bone health. To keep the blood healthy, they produce a hormone called *erythropoietin (erith-ro-po-eaten)*, which fuels the production of red blood cells in bone marrow. This helps the body prevent *anemia*, or a low red blood count.

To maintain bone health, the kidneys transform and "activate" vitamin D that's obtained from both diet and sun exposure. Vitamin D is responsible for preserving bone, heart, and total body health. Unfortunately, many of us in this country are deficient in this important vitamin. Proper supplementation of this essential vitamin is crucial, and will be discussed further in Chapters 5 and 8 (see pages 70 and 111).

THE STAGES OF KIDNEY DISEASE

Now you know that the kidneys perform a range of essential functions. When kidney disease develops, though, the function of these organs begins to diminish.

Earlier in this chapter, you learned that kidney function is measured in terms of how well the glomeruli—the tiny filters in the kidney—clean the blood. Physicians express this in terms of the *glomerular filtration rate* (GFR). The GFR is easily calculated from a blood test that measures your level of creatinine (a waste material that results from muscle metabolism) and other factors such as age, gender, and size. A normal GFR is greater than 90 mL/min (90 milliliters per minute). As the GFR falls, your kidneys have a lesser ability to filter out waste. Doctors also get a sense of how poorly kidney function may be based on the appearance of the kidneys as seen on medical imaging such as a kidney ultrasound. The presence of protein and/or blood in the urine can also be a sign of damage being done to the kidneys or of a potential problem that can cause kidney damage.

Based on the factors discussed above—GFR and kidney damage—physicians determine the stage of an individual's kidney disease. Table 1.1 briefly describes these five stages.

Table 1.1. The Five Stages of Chronic Kidney Disease

Stage	Description	Glomerular Filtration Rate (GFR)
Stage 1	Kidney damage with normal or high GFR. In this stage, protein is being spilled into the urine.	90 mL/min or higher
Stage 2	Kidney damage with a mild decrease in GFR.	60–89 mL/min
Stage 3	Kidney damage with a moderate decrease in GFR.	30–59 mL/min
Stage 4	Kidney damage with a severe decrease in GFR.	15–29 mL/min
Stage 5	Kidney failure. (At this stage, patients often need to start kidney dialysis.)	Less than 15 mL/min

Doctors often start talking to a patient about dialysis when kidney disease is in Stage 4 and the GFR is between 15 and 29 mL/min. Kidney dialysis becomes necessary at some point in Stage 5, usually when the GFR is less than 10 mL/min and there is 10 percent or less kidney function remaining. However, doctors make the determination to begin dialysis based not just on numbers, but also on the individual's overall health. Some people with 10 percent kidney function do not need to start dialysis right away, but, instead, are closely monitored by their doctor. In other individuals, the presence of medical conditions such as edema (discussed on page 12) make it necessary to begin dialysis sooner than expected.

Stage 5 of chronic kidney disease is also referred to as *end stage renal disease (ESRD), end stage kidney disease, renal failure,* or *kidney failure.* In the next section, you'll learn about the symptoms and medical problems that are likely to occur during this stage.

SIGNS THAT DIALYSIS MAY BE NECESSARY

Because the kidneys play a part in so many vital processes in the body, their failure results in a variety of signs, symptoms, and health conditions. Some of these conditions may be very noticeable to you or the people around you, and some may be revealed only through medical testing. To understand the need for dialysis, it's important to know a little about what happens in the body when the kidneys no longer do their job. Keep in mind that, as explained above, doctors take a number of factors into account before recommending dialysis. Your kidney doctor, or *nephrologist (nef-ralla-gist),* will consider not only your degree of kidney function, but also whether you are tired all the time, whether you have an appetite, or whether you have other symptoms which indicate that your body needs help.

Uremia

The chief function of the kidneys is to filter poisons out of the blood so that they can be eliminated from the body. When the kidneys can no longer adequately filter the blood, you experience a condition known as *uremia (your-eem-eeya),* due to the daily buildup of over one hundred uremic toxins.

Uremic symptoms can occur quickly or slowly, depending on the time it takes for your kidneys to reach the level of about 10 percent or less functioning. Some examples of these uremic symptoms include nausea, vomiting, and an altered or metallic taste. Another common symptom is *pruritus (pru-rye-tis),* or itching. This is not a local skin irritation; it is a major body itch. People often say that their whole body itches from the inside out. Although pruritis can be caused by the accumulation of toxins, it can also be caused by very high phosphorus levels. This is further discussed in Chapter 4, where the specific blood tests concerning dialysis are reviewed.

Other uremic symptoms can include decreased appetite, muscle cramping, hiccups, confusion, and/or problems with sleep. Remember that you can have any or all of the above symptoms, and that these symptoms can be subtle. You may have difficulty sleeping or concentrating, or you may just feel sick and tired of being constantly "sick and tired." Any of these symptoms can be an indication that dialysis should be started.

Heart and Blood Vessel Problems

Uremia, discussed above, has very widespread effects, and one of the most serious consequences can be heart disease. That's one reason why people with kidney disease are followed so closely by their doctor. When the heart is affected by uremia, there is an increased risk of developing *coronary artery disease (CAD)*—narrowing of the blood vessels that supply blood and oxygen to the heart—or of experiencing a worsening of existing CAD. Over time, the heart's ability to perform its primary task of pumping blood to the rest of the body can be reduced, as can its ability to "relax" between contractions. (You'll learn more about this on page 12.) Other complications of kidney disease, including anemia and bone disease, can also affect your heart.

The uremic toxins can also cause inflammation of the lining surrounding the heart, called the *pericardium (perry-card-ee-um)*. The pericardium surrounds the heart in much the same way that a bed sheet covers a mattress. Inflammation of this lining can develop into *uremic pericarditis,* a life-threatening emergency that requires immediate dialysis.

Anemia

As explained earlier, the kidneys produce a hormone that stimulates the bone marrow to produce the proper number of red blood cells. In advanced kidney disease, the kidneys no longer make the hormone that says to the bone marrow, "I need more red blood cells." This leads to the development of *anemia,* or an insufficient number of red blood cells. Since the primary function of these cells is to carry oxygen throughout the body, anemia causes oxygen deficiency, which results in symptoms such as fatigue and weakness. When kidney function diminishes to the point that dialysis is needed, these symptoms can be worsened by uremia.

Problems with Fluid Control and Swelling

Physicians may advise patients to consider dialysis when the body is unable to get rid of extra fluids, which can build up in the tissues despite the aggressive use of diuretics (water pills) such as Lasix (furosemide) and Zaroxolyn (metolazone). Doctors refer to this accumulation of fluids as *fluid overload* or *volume overload*.

Fluids can build up in the body due to kidney failure itself, due to heart problems, or due to a combination of the two. The basic function of the left ventricle of the heart is to pump blood to the rest of the body. The heart works in concert with the kidneys to eliminate extra sodium and fluid in order to keep the body in balance. When the kidneys can't get rid of the extra fluid and/or the heart becomes either too weak to pump well (called *systolic failure)* or too stiff to relax (called *diastolic failure)*, the fluid isn't able to be effectively eliminated by the kidneys, and it builds up in the body. It's important to remember that kidney failure and heart problems are so intertwined that it is impossible to separate one from the other. The condition that exists when both kidneys and heart are dysfunctional is referred to as *cardiorenal syndrome (CRS)*.

Common symptoms of fluid overload can include swollen legs caused by *edema*, or excess fluid trapped in the body's tissues; fluid in the lungs; or *congestive heart failure (CHF)*, a condition in which the heart cannot pump enough blood to the rest of the body. Some people gain fluid weight in their abdominal area and complain that fluid buildup in the belly is causing waistbands to fit too tightly. This is different from an expanded waistline that results from obesity; fluid buildup is a process that can happen in a matter of days, whereas weight due to overeating accumulates over a period of weeks. Often, people complain of massive weight gain because of significant fluid retention that requires higher and higher doses of diuretics. In many cases, these diuretics can be a double-edged sword; they can help the body get rid of the extra fluid, but they can also make the kidneys work harder and adversely affect kidney function.

In very advanced kidney disease, kidney function can be so poor that no amount of diuretic works. When a doctor suggests dialysis, the person has probably experienced multiple hospital admissions for volume overload and/or CHF requiring diuretics. In this situation, dialysis can help by not only filtering out toxins but also removing excess fluids through a process called *ultrafiltration (ultra-fil-tray-shun)*, which you'll learn more about later in the book. CHF and fluid overload are the most common causes of admission and readmission to the hospital.

Abnormal Blood Work

From an earlier discussion (see page 9), you know that a physician's recommendation to use dialysis is partly based on the GFR, which shows the degree to which the kidneys are functioning. But nephrologists actually consider other blood work results, as well.

One marker that doctors consider closely is the level of albumin. Albumin is the most abundant protein in the blood and has many important functions, such as preventing fluid from leaking out of blood vessels, nourishing tissues, and transporting important substances like vitamins throughout the body. A normal level of albumin is considered 4 mg/dL (milligrams per deciliter). When the albumin level drops, it is a sign that the individual has kidney disease, is not eating enough protein, and/or has inflammation—a characteristic of kidney disease that affects not only the kidneys, but other organs, as well. Keep in mind, though, that although a single test of serum (blood) albumin is valuable, doctors like to "trend" laboratory results by comparing them from one month to the next. (You'll learn more about albumin on page 57 of Chapter 4.)

Another indication that dialysis is needed is a high potassium level. Healthy kidneys remove excess potassium from the bloodstream, keeping levels between 3.5 and 5 mEq/L (milliequivalents per liter). When kidney dysfunction prevents the control of potassium, the result is *hyperkalemia (hyper-ka-leemia)*, or high blood levels of potassium. An excess of potassium can cause an abnormal heart rhythm, called an *arrhythmia*. Physicians generally measure the potassium level through blood work and also obtain an *electrocardiogram*, or *EKG*, to evaluate the effect of the potassium on the heart. A very high potassium level coupled with certain EKG changes can indicate an urgent need for dialysis treatments.

Another indication that dialysis may be needed is the *blood urea nitrogen (BUN)*, test. When proteins are broken down in the body, the liver takes the waste products, which include nitrogen, to make a substance known as urea. The urea is transported via the bloodstream from the liver to the kidneys, where it is filtered from the blood for elimination from the body. When the kidneys lose their filtering abilities, the BUN level rises. A normal range is generally considered between 6 and 20 mg/dL (milligrams per deciliter). Although the BUN test, in and of itself, is not an indication to begin dialysis, the results may be taken into consideration along with the other blood work and health conditions described above.

HOW LONG CAN YOU STAY ON DIALYSIS?

When people begin dialysis or consider the possible need for this treatment, most ask questions such as, "How long can I live on dialysis?" or "Will I have to remain on dialysis for the rest of my life?"

Once kidney disease progresses to a certain level, dialysis is needed to perform some of the functions that can no longer be carried out by these vital organs. The good news is that dialysis is much more effective than it was when it was first introduced decades ago, and that some people have been on dialysis for thirty years or more without getting a transplant. How well your body does on this treatment depends on several factors, including your general health aside from the kidney disease; whether you receive good quality dialysis and medical care; and whether you follow your diet, exercise, and treatment prescriptions. The more informed you become and the more active role you take in your own care, the better you will do on dialysis. That's why this book was written—to give you the information, practical advice, and complementary options that will help you deal as successfully as possible with your treatment.

In answering the question, "Will I have to remain on dialysis for the rest of my life?" it's important to bring up the option of a kidney transplant. Many people have been able to get off dialysis by obtaining a kidney from a living donor or the national waiting list. If your GFR is less than 20 mL/min, in addition to discussing dialysis, a transplant evaluation should be considered. (For more information on transplants, see Chapter 11.)

IN CONCLUSION

Doctors generally consider a number of factors before recommending dialysis. They carefully review the results of medical tests that indicate the kidneys' level of function, and—as long as there is no urgent need for immediately dialysis—they also consider how you are feeling and how kidney disease is affecting your general well-being. But the decision to start dialysis is really only the beginning of a journey that will involve further decisions. Often, you can choose the type of dialysis that you will have and decide whether you have the dialysis at home or at a hospital or other dialysis center. These choices are important since they will have a significant effect on both your physical health and the quality of your day-to-day life. Chapter 2 takes you further on your journey by exploring the different types of dialysis that may be available to you.

2

What Are Your Dialysis Options?

In Chapter 1, you read about the "when" of dialysis—the different conditions and indications that mean it's time to start treatment. Now you may be wondering what dialysis is and how it works. This chapter addresses the different types of dialysis available, providing the information you need to understand your options. Before we "talk tech," though, we need to discuss something more important: having hope and belief in yourself throughout the adjustment period and beyond.

THE ADJUSTMENT PERIOD

I am not going to lie to you. Dialysis, no matter what type you choose, is a life-changing experience. The transition can be difficult, but it is not impossible. Both your body and your emotions will take some time to adjust.

Every person is different, of course, and will have a unique adjustment period. Not everyone takes to the same type of dialysis; that is why there are so many different options available. One of the "secrets" to surviving and thriving on dialysis has to do with understanding which *modality* (method) works for you.

One question that is often asked concerning dialysis is, "How will it make me feel?" People who choose peritoneal dialysis, home-based therapies, or even nocturnal hemodialysis usually do well from the start because these modalities are gentler and allow the body more time to adjust to the process. Perhaps more important, these forms of dialysis give people a greater sense of control.

From my experience, people on in-center three-times-a-week dialysis can respond in three different ways. About a third of people who start standard in-center hemodialysis take to it like a fish to water. They have been sick so long that they have forgotten what it's like to feel "normal." Now, they have pep in their step, and they feel like they have regained part of their life.

The second group of people feels "worn-out" after dialysis. They report feeling good on their non-dialysis days, but after dialysis, they may need to go home and rest. Some are better after they sleep for a few hours, but many are exhausted for the rest of the day.

The third group of people feels bad all of the time. On their dialysis days, on their non-dialysis days, they just aren't well, and dialysis makes everything worse. They tend to skip treatments, and can end up going to the hospital for urgent dialysis. Again, for the most part, I am talking about in-center three-times-a-week dialysis therapy.

Why do some people feel so bad on dialysis? After all, doesn't dialysis actually relieve the physical stress caused by the buildup of excess toxins and fluids? Well, recall that your kidney filters your blood twenty-four hours a day, seven days a week. That is 168 hours a week of continuous filtering. A typical in-center dialysis treatment is four hours long, three times a week. This means that dialysis tries to do in twelve hours what kidneys normally do on a continuous basis over the course of a week. Besides filtering toxins, dialysis removes built-up fluids—fluids that have accumulated over a period of days—in just four hours. This places a strain on the body, and some people just don't tolerate it. I want to emphasize, however, that many people do well on in-center dialysis. Everyone is different, and the dialysis that is best for one person is not necessarily the right choice for someone else. Again, that is why understanding all of your dialysis options is so important.

So far, we have talked about the physical toll that dialysis takes on some people, but these physical difficulties can take an emotional and spiritual toll, as well. That's why it's so important not only to keep your head in the game when starting dialysis, but also to not lose hope during the adjustment period and to believe that you can do well. A positive attitude is so essential that it needs to be talked about right here, right now, before we discuss the technical aspects of dialysis. Before you read any further, put this book down, take a deep breath, and say, "I can do this." Repeat it again and again. Believe in what you're saying, and believe in yourself. Also understand that you're not in this alone. You have a whole team of people there for you. A mentor of mine once told me, "If you can conceive and believe, then you can achieve." The same goes for starting dialysis. Now, let's talk logistics.

THE MODALITY REVIEW

For anyone who needs to make a decision about dialysis treatment, nothing is more valuable than a modality review. During this review, you sit down with a health professional—usually a trained nurse with a specialty in dialysis—who explains the dialysis process and the options that are available to you. These reviews are often held in a dialysis unit so that you can see what the unit looks like and what a typical hemodialysis session entails, and perhaps even talk to someone on dialysis to get an invaluable personal perspective of the process. Note that although modality reviews take place in dedicated units, they cover all types of dialysis, including hemodialysis (HD) and peritoneal dialysis (PD), in-center treatments and home-based treatments. If you choose a home-based dialysis therapy, further instruction will be provided, including videos as well as one-on-one instruction and interaction with other dialysis patients and their significant others.

Many dialysis units and comprehensive care clinics provide group classes in addition to the individual modality reviews. One popular option is a group session in which a medical professional not only reviews the different types of dialysis, but also provides information concerning diet and nutrition, the importance of the dialysis access (you'll learn more about that in Chapter 3), and other relevant topics, including ones that may be specific to you and your family member or significant other.

All dialysis centers can provide modality reviews. Some do so for every new dialysis patient, and some, only when a patient requests one. If a review isn't automatically provided for you, speak to your doctor about setting one up.

How Does a Hemodialysis Machine Work?

Hemodialysis is the most common treatment for kidney failure. This chapter explains that there are three "modes" of hemodialysis—standard three-times-a-week in-center dialysis, nocturnal dialysis, and home dialysis. Regardless of when and where you have this treatment, your blood is filtered via a dialysis machine. How does this machine work? You are about to find out.

As you'll learn in Chapter 3, an *access* that's created in your body provides an entryway to your bloodstream. Tubing is connected from your access to the dialysis machine. One tube carries your blood into the machine, and another carries the dialyzed blood out of the machine and back into your bloodstream.

When your blood enters the dialysis machine, it is carried through the machine's *dialyzer,* which is a special filter. (See Figure 2.1.) Your blood runs one way through this filter, while a chemical solution called a *dialysate* runs in the opposite direction. The dialysate is specially designed to draw toxins out of the bloodstream. The blood and dialysate never touch, but are separated by a semipermeable membrane. Through the process of *diffusion*—in which dissolved chemicals move from an area of high concentration (in this case, the blood) to one of lower concentration (the dialysate)—excess waste products and toxins, which are small in size, pass through the membrane into the dialysate. Through a process called *ultrafiltration,* excess fluid is also removed from the blood. Together, these actions duplicate the filtering process that takes place in healthy kidneys. In fact, the dialyzer is sometimes referred to as an "artificial kidney," although it does not do all that a functioning kidney can do. Dialyzers are available in several sizes so that the right size can be used for each patient. When a patient first begins dialysis, usually a smaller filter is used. If the blood work shows that more waste products have to be removed, a larger dialyzer may be introduced.

The dialysis machine is designed to carefully regulate the filtering process. It monitors the rate of blood flow outside your body, it helps normalize the blood's levels of minerals and electrolytes, and it controls the temperature and proper mixture of the dialysate. If any of these important factors go out of range, the machine lets your dialysis team know by sounding an alarm. The machine also signals if your blood pressure is too high or too low so that adjustments can be made. It even signals when the dialysis session is over.

When your blood has been filtered through the dialysis machine, it is carried back into your body. The dialysate—which now contains the toxins, wastes, and excess fluids removed from the blood—leaves the dialyzer and is flushed down the drain.

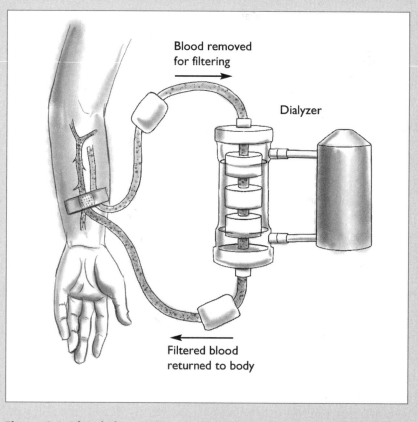

Figure 2.1. Blood Flow Between Hemodialysis Patient and Dialyzer.
During hemodialysis, blood passes through the machine's dialyzer, which draws waste products and excess fluid out of the blood and into the dialysis solution. The filtered blood then re-enters the body.

YOUR DIALYSIS OPTIONS

When I was undergoing my fellowship training, the options for those starting dialysis were limited. They included regular *hemodialysis (hemoe-dye-ala-cis)*, or HD, which involved going to a designated outpatient dialysis center three times a week; and *peritoneal dialysis (pera-ta-neal dye-ala-cis)*, or PD, which could be performed at home. Since that time, other viable options have become available, specifically, *nocturnal dialysis*, or ND, and *home hemodialysis*, or home HD. Below, you'll learn more about each of these options.

Hemodialysis (HD)

Hemodialysis (HD) is the process by which your blood is cleaned and filtered through a dialysis machine. The blood is removed from the body via a dialysis *access*—a dialysis catheter, a graft, or a fistula, which you'll learn about in Chapter 3—and then travels through the machine, where it is filtered and cleaned. It is then returned to your body. (For a closer look at the dialysis machine and what it does, see the inset on pages 20 to 21.)

In the United States, hemodialysis is usually performed during a relatively short session in a specialized facility. This is called *in-center dialysis*. But it can also be performed in a dialysis facility overnight, as *nocturnal dialysis (ND)*, or in your own home, as *home hemodialysis (home HD)*. Let's look at each of these options in turn.

In-Center Dialysis

In-center dialysis treatments occur three times a week, usually on a Monday-Wednesday-Friday or Tuesday-Thursday-Saturday schedule. The duration of each treatment is around four hours, although it can vary depending upon the individual's size and muscle mass, as well as how efficiently the blood is being cleaned by the dialysis as determined by blood work. (You'll learn about blood work in Chapter 4.)

The upside of this form of treatment is that your dialysis is taken care of by trained professionals who have a great deal of experience in using the equipment and monitoring the patient throughout the process. Another positive aspect is that because the treatments occur in a dedicated center, you don't need to turn a room in your house into a "dialysis room." Also, most centers offer a degree of flexibility regarding the time of the treatment. They may, for instance, provide sessions early in the morning, in the afternoon, and even in the evening for those who work during the day.

The downside of in-center hemodialysis is that once your schedule is chosen, you have to adhere to the facility's timetable. Also, the three-times-a-week sessions provide at most twelve hours of dialysis each week, so fluids and toxins can build up quite a bit between treatments. This means that you must follow a strict diet and, in most cases, take several medications to minimize toxic buildup, fluid overload, and other problems. During treatments, a large amount of excess fluids may have to be removed in a fairly short period of time, which can be tough on your body. (You'll learn more about that in Chapter 6.) Nevertheless, standard hemodialysis works well for many people.

Nocturnal Dialysis (ND)

As the name indicates, nocturnal dialysis (ND) is performed overnight—usually for six to eight hours a night, three nights a week—at a dedicated dialysis center. It doesn't take a great mathematician to see that this provides more treatment than daytime in-center dialysis. It can, in fact, double your dialysis time. While this involves a very regimented schedule and requires you to spend three nights a week away from home, those on nocturnal dialysis often feel a lot better, have less problems with fluid overload, and need to follow fewer dietary restrictions than people who have standard hemodialysis. People who have switched from standard HD to nocturnal HD often say that their appetite and general sense of well-being have improved. Because fluid weight is removed over a longer period of time, their bodies have more time to adjust during treatments. They also require fewer medications for the treatment of blood pressure—and any reduction in the number of medications is a good thing. I do weekly rounds on a nocturnal dialysis shift, and for the most part, these patients report feeling better than they did on standard HD.

Who is a good candidate for nocturnal dialysis? One can argue that anyone is a candidate for nocturnal dialysis, as every individual would benefit from it. That being said, those who weigh more or who gain a large amount of fluid weight in between treatments often find that nocturnal dialysis is a good choice, because the removal of fluid is more gradual. Anyone who switches to nocturnal HD just has to understand that it's necessary to spend three nights a week at the dialysis center. Some people adjust quickly, but some have trouble dealing with the "noises" of the dialysis machine or, for some other reason, find it difficult to sleep away from home.

Home Hemodialysis (Home HD)

As the name implies, home hemodialysis (home HD) is performed in your own home. It is similar to in-center HD, but the dialysis machine is much smaller, about the size of a small refrigerator, and you (or a family member or friend) assume the role of the dialysis technician. To use this therapy at home, you will need a designated area of your house that is clean, safe, and secure.

Home HD treatments are generally shorter but more frequent than those provided in standard in-center dialysis. It is common to have four or five treatments a week, each of which ranges from two and a half to three and a half hours, depending on your body size and muscle mass. (The average is five weekly treatments of three hours each.)

Many people who opt for home HD are already on in-center dialysis. Whether or not you're now having in-center treatments, you will need several weeks of training, during which you will learn how to:

- prepare equipment and supplies

- place the needle in the vascular access

- program and monitor the machine

- check blood pressure and pulse

- keep records of the treatments

- clean the equipment and the room where dialysis is performed

- order supplies

- collect monthly blood samples and send them to the lab

- use aseptic technique to minimize the risk of infection

If you are considering home HD, it is strongly recommended that you bring a "helper"—a family member or friend—to the training sessions so that you'll have a great support person who is also trained in the mechanics of home HD. There will then be two dialysis technicians in your home. Most clinics, in fact, *require* a helper on home HD. Even if you are the only one being trained in the technical aspects of dialysis, it is strongly recommended that someone else be close by during your home dialysis treatments.

One of the most common questions people ask is, "Can *anyone* do home HD?" The quick answer to this is if you can operate a car, you can do home HD. There is going to be a learning curve, but that's why the training takes several weeks. Some aspects of the treatment may be trickier than others. For instance, one of the biggest hurdles for most people is learning to "access" their own dialysis access using aseptic techniques. (You'll learn about this in Chapter 3.) Remember what we talked about in the beginning of the chapter? If you believe in yourself and in your ability to master dialysis, you will be able to do it!

Understand that you will not be in this alone. In addition to your nephrologist, you will have your home HD nurse, who will be your teacher, support, and friend. She will be there for you, and if you have questions or run into trouble, someone will be available twenty-four hours a day. (To learn more about your dialysis team, see the inset on page 28.)

Despite the fact that people who do home HD have to learn new skills and be responsible for their own dialysis, those who practice it highly recommend it. They say that they have more lifestyle freedom and flexibility. While before they had to adjust their lives around their dialysis, they find that with home HD, they can, in fact, adjust their dialysis around their lives. And because they are able to perform dialysis several times a week, toxins and fluids have less time to accumulate, making them feel a whole lot better.

Peritoneal Dialysis (PD)

Peritoneal dialysis (PD) is very different from hemodialysis in that rather than using an artificial filter, it utilizes the peritoneal membrane, which is the natural semipermeable membrane that lines your abdominal cavity, or belly. In this case, your dialysis access is a catheter called a *peritoneal dialysis catheter,* or PD catheter. A dextrose-based solution, called a *dialysate,* is infused into your belly through the access. The solution serves to pull out not only the toxins that build up in the body, but also any excess fluid, so that like a hemodialysis machine, it performs both dialysis and ultrafiltration. The fluid is then drained from the abdomen, removing the toxins and built-up fluids. The amount of fluid removed is controlled by the type of solution used. Solutions that contain more dextrose generally remove greater volumes of fluid.

There are two forms of PD. In *continuous ambulatory peritoneal dialysis (CAPD),* on an average of three or four times a day, you fill your abdomen with the dialysate. Then, after a prescribed *dwell time*—which can range from two to four hours, depending on your specific dialysis prescription—you drain the fluid into a bag. The amount of fluid infused each time is about two liters (approximately two quarts), although this, too, can vary. The reason this is called "ambulatory" is that during the "dwell time," you can walk around with the solution in your belly. This system does not use a machine, and the fluid that is drained out can be emptied down the household drain. It does not contain any blood.

After you become comfortable with manual exchanges, you will probably be given the option of switching to *automated peritoneal dialysis,* or *APD,* which uses a machine known as a *cycler.* The cycler can be used at night while you are sleeping and is programmed to perform several exchanges over a defined period of time, usually eight to ten hours. Some people have difficulty sleeping through the exchanges because the cycler beeps loudly when there is a problem, or because they don't feel comfortable sleeping with a belly full of fluid. The majority of people on PD, though, prefer using the cycler because it frees up their days and makes it unnecessary to perform manual exchanges. Just like the fluid drained through the ambulatory method, this fluid can be emptied down the household drain.

Like any home-based form of dialysis, home PD means that you will need a designated area of your home that is clean, safe, and secure. It also means that you will have to learn some new skills. Usually, people begin by learning how to do manual exchanges in a dialysis center. This can take a few weeks. Later, if they choose to use a cycler, they are trained in automated PD. During training, you will be taught how to:

- prepare equipment and supplies

- perform the manual exchanges, including accessing the peritoneal dialysis catheter, infusing the fluid, and draining the fluid

- program and troubleshoot the cycler (if you switch to automated PD)

- check blood pressure and pulse

- keep records of treatments, including weight gains and losses and the amount of fluid drained

- clean the equipment and the area where dialysis is performed

- order supplies

- use aseptic technique to minimize the risk of infection

There are some key points you need to be aware of concerning PD. First, this is something you can do on your own. While it can be beneficial to have a helper trained in PD, it is not as necessary as it is with home HD. Second, the amount of dialysis you need to do really depends on the amount of residual (remaining) kidney function you have. Although you have advanced kidney disease, in many cases, there is still 5 to 10 percent residual kidney function, which can make a big difference. The more residual kidney function you have, the less PD you will need.

HOW DO YOU DECIDE WHICH TREATMENT IS RIGHT FOR YOU?

You now know a bit more about the different dialysis options that are available to you, as well as each option's pros and cons. The next question that usually comes up is, "How do I decide which one is for me?" Well, sometimes an option immediately appeals to you, and sometimes you have to systematically consider the pros and cons of each treatment to decide which option is the best fit.

One of the biggest choices you have to make concerns whether you want to go to a dedicated treatment center or pursue a home-based therapy. If you choose in-center treatment, your dialysis time will be dictated

Members of the Dialysis Team

No matter what type of dialysis treatment you choose, you will be interacting with many of the same team members. On dialysis, a team approach is vital, so let's review the players.

The Nephrologist. The nephrologist, or kidney specialist, is the "coach" of the team. Along with you, she directs the other players involved. If you choose in-center dialysis, you will likely see your doctor, another doctor from her practice, or an advanced practitioner (a nurse practitioner or physician's assistant) on a once-a-week basis. If you are pursuing a home-based therapy, you may see the doctor during a scheduled visit once a month.

The Physician's Assistant (PA) or Nurse Practitioner (NP). The PA and/or NP works with the nephrologist. If you have in-center dialysis, you will probably see this team member once a week.

The Dietitian. The dietitian is one of the most important members of your team. Given the many dietary modifications that someone on dialysis must follow, the input of a dietitian is invaluable. In many in-patient centers, the dietitian meets with the dialysis patient at least once a month to discuss nutrition issues and review monthly blood work. (For more information concerning your monthly labs, please turn to Chapter 4. For information on dietary considerations, see Chapter 9.)

The Case Manager. A case manager is a nurse or social worker who helps in the planning, coordination, and monitoring of a patient's medical care. During the course of dialysis treatment, many issues can arise concerning insurance, getting necessary medications, and other aspects of therapy. It is the case manager's job to work out these problems so that you will receive the care you need.

The Dialysis Nurse. Whether you are receiving in-center dialysis or you choose to learn home care skills, a dialysis nurse is vitally important. If you are dialyzing at an inpatient center, you will see the nurse frequently. Many times, in addition to supervising your dialysis sessions, these nurses become trusted friends and confidants.

The Dialysis Technician. A dialysis technician is specially trained for in-center hemodialysis care. Along with the nurse, she operates and maintains dialysis equipment and closely monitors each dialysis session.

by a fixed schedule; your session will begin at a certain time and end at a certain time, with the specific schedule depending in part on the time slots available at the dialysis center. This can make it difficult to meet work and family obligations. The upside, of course, is that you don't have to take care of your own dialysis. A trained team of medical professionals provides a clean environment and maintained equipment, runs and monitors the dialysis, and performs and interprets the lab tests.

The big advantage of home-based therapies, including PD and home HD, is that there is so much flexibility. This option takes into account work and family schedules and can accommodate a busy lifestyle. The downside? You are the driving force behind your dialysis. Yes, you will have a support team available in terms of your doctor, your dialysis nurse, and, perhaps, your family, but you will be responsible for performing your own treatments. If you choose PD, you will be doing this on a daily basis. If you choose home HD, you will probably have four or five sessions a week, with the times dependent on your schedule.

There is, of course, another important consideration: Which dialysis option is better for you physically? Realize that any type of dialysis places physical stress on the body. Standard in-center dialysis tends to place the most stress on the body because of the amount of filtering and fluid removal that has to be performed in such a short period of time. Home HD (with its frequent, shorter sessions) and nocturnal HD (which doubles standard dialysis time) tend to be better tolerated because the body has more time to adjust. PD is very well tolerated by most people for the same reason. That being said, the physical toll of a specific form of dialysis is different for different people. Your goal is to find the one that works best for you.

In general, home HD, nocturnal HD, and PD also allow for a better quality of life. Less blood pressure medication is often needed, and the amount of phosphorus binders may also be reduced. Moreover, these modes of dialysis can promote better appetite and a greater overall sense of well-being. Again, this is not true for everyone, but it is true for many people.

If your doctor says that you are free to choose any form of dialysis that you prefer, but you're having trouble making your decision, consider the following factors:

- **Having equipment in your home.** Would it bother you to see a dialysis machine and other medical equipment in your home—possibly, in your bedroom?

- **Sleeping.** Can you sleep anywhere at any time, or would you have trouble getting a good night's sleep while attached to a hemodialysis machine or a cycler?

- **Dietary limitations.** In-center hemodialysis imposes the most dietary limitations; nocturnal HD, the least. What kind of dietary restrictions are you willing to live with each day?

- **Limitations on evening activities.** Using a PD cycler can shorten your evenings because of the longer treatment time. Nocturnal hemodialysis can also affect evening activities, although only a few nights a week. Will this interfere with time spent with family and friends?

- **Child care.** Do you have young children at home? Will someone be able to care for them if you have treatment in a dedicated center?

- **Medications.** In-center HD usually means taking the most pills—an average of nineteen pills a day—to help control the level of toxins in the blood between treatments. Nocturnal HD usually involves the least amount of medication. How many pills are you willing to take each day?

- **Employment.** If you have a job, how will your treatments affect your work life? Will you be able to take off the time needed for in-center dialysis or other daytime treatments?

- **Getting to treatments.** Will you have trouble getting to a dialysis center for treatment? Is there a good center near you, and is affordable transportation available?

- **Being responsible for your own care.** I've already said that anyone who drives a car can learn the skills necessary for home dialysis, but you will have to not only learn these skills but also maintain aseptic conditions, keep medical supplies on hand, and be diligent and disciplined in your self-care. Are you comfortable with the idea of being responsible for your own dialysis, or would you prefer to place your treatments in the hands of a medical team?

Switching From One Type of Dialysis to Another

An important question that sometimes arises is: "Can I switch to another type of dialysis?" This most often comes up when someone started on in-hospital hemodialysis because of medical necessity. She may have remained on dialysis for a period of time and become more medically stable. Now she wants to explore other options.

Usually, it *is* possible to switch to another type of treatment, but the options depend on the individual's medical condition, support system, and capabilities. In my own practice, one person began on in-hospital hemodialysis and transitioned to home HD. With the flexibility brought by home care, she now has a new lease on life. Another person began on hospital HD and transitioned to peritoneal dialysis. She, too, is feeling better and experiencing greater quality of life. So don't think that once you select a treatment mode, you have to stick with it forever. Especially if you are willing and able to learn new skills, other dialysis options are usually open to you.

As you see, there are a lot of considerations. Just remember that if the treatment option you choose doesn't work for you or if your needs change over time, you will probably be able to switch from one type of treatment to another. (See the inset above.)

IN CONCLUSION

This chapter has provided you with a brief overview of the different types of dialysis available. In general, the more dialysis you get, the better you will feel. By better controlling the buildup of toxins and fluids, frequent dialysis minimizes ups and downs and helps avoid the wiped-out feeling many people experience after treatment. This is why people generally do better when they choose nocturnal HD, home HD, or peritoneal dialysis. Home-based therapies have the added advantage of offering flexible schedules that can interfere less with work, play, and family. But everyone's needs and situation are different, and only you can pick the dialysis option that's right for you.

Regardless of the type of dialysis you choose, some type of *access* will be created—an entryway to your bloodstream (for hemodialysis) or your peritoneum (for peritoneal dialysis). This access is so important that it is the focus of Chapter 3.

3

ℐhe Importance of the Dialysis Access

As I stated in the last chapter, your *dialysis access*—a specially created entryway into your bloodstream (for hemodialysis) or your abdominal cavity (for peritoneal dialysis)—is your lifeline. No matter the type of dialysis you are using, a well-functioning access will allow you to get the treatments that you need to live and maintain quality of life, and a poorly functioning access can literally cost you your life. That's why this chapter tells you what each type of access is; how it is created; how long it takes to heal and, in some cases, "mature" before use; and how you can best take care of it. If you are going to have a hemodialysis (HD) access created in the future, this chapter even tells you how to protect the arm that will be used for the access so that it will remain strong and healthy.

The pages that follow first look at the three types of access used for hemodialysis. They then examine the single access used for peritoneal dialysis (PD). (For a quick reference to the different access types, see Table 3.1.) Finally, the chapter provides important guidelines for taking care of your access.

ACCESS FOR HEMODIALYSIS

Three types of access are used for hemodialysis. The preferred option is the fistula. It works the best and is least prone to problems. The second best option is the graft. Catheters are the third and least ideal option, and are usually used only on a temporary basis until a fistula or graft can be created through surgery and allowed to heal and mature. The

Table 3.1. Types of Dialysis Access

For Hemodialysis	
Name of Access	**Fistula**
What Is It?	A surgically created direct connection between an artery and a vein.
Where Is It Placed?	Usually placed in the forearm of the nondominant arm. Sometimes, in the upper arm or even the leg.
Considerations:	• Best overall performance for hemodialysis access.
	• Takes two months or more to heal and mature after surgery.
	• Allows for good blood flow during dialysis.
	• Makes repeated needle insertion easier.
	• Lasts longer than other types of dialysis access—in some cases, for several decades.
	• Less prone to infection and clotting than other types of dialysis access.
Name of Access	**Graft**
What Is It?	A surgically created indirect connection between an artery and a vein via an artificial tube placed between them.
Where Is It Placed?	Usually placed in the forearm of the nondominant arm. Sometimes, in the upper arm or even the leg.
Considerations:	• Can be used within two to four weeks after surgery.
	• Allows for good blood flow, but not as good as that of fistula.
	• Typically used when patients have small, weak veins that won't permit a fistula.
	• Allows repeated needle insertion.
	• More prone to infection and clotting than a fistula.
	• Doesn't last as long as a fistula, but in some cases, can last for several years.

catheter is always used when someone is urgently started on HD in the hospital because of acute kidney failure.

For Hemodialysis

Name of Access	**Catheter**
What Is It?	A surgical attachment of a flexible tube to a vein or artery.
Where Is It Placed?	• A *jugular catheter* is inserted in the jugular vein on the side of the neck.
	• A *subclavian catheter* is placed in the subclavian vein under the collarbone.
	• A *femoral catheter* is placed in the large femoral vein in the leg, near the groin.
Considerations:	• Can be used immediately after insertion.
	• Typically used on emergency basis or when waiting for fistula or graft to heal.
	• Can be easily removed and replaced.
	• Does not allow good blood flow during dialysis.
	• More prone to infection than fistula or graft, but proper care can reduce the risk.
	• Not ideal as permanent access.

For Peritoneal Dialysis

Name of Access	**Catheter**
What Is It?	A small, flexible tube implanted in the abdomen.
Where Is It Placed?	Always inserted in the abdominal cavity.
Considerations:	• Is the only access option when using peritoneal dialysis.
	• Can be used two or three weeks after surgery, although most doctors wait four weeks.
	• Typically lasts several years before needing replacement.
	• More prone to infection than fistula or graft, but proper care can reduce the risk.

The Hemodialysis Fistula

As explained in Chapter 1, nephrologists usually begin talking to a patient about dialysis when his kidney disease has progressed to Stage 4 and the GFR is between 15 and 29 mL/min. At this point, there is generally 15 to 29 percent kidney function. One reason that doctors want to discuss dialysis before it is medically necessary is that time is needed to surgically create an access and allow it to heal and *mature*—that is, to get big enough in size and develop well enough to be used in dialysis. This is especially true of the fistula, which represents the gold standard for dialysis access and takes at least two months—sometimes longer—to mature before dialysis can begin.

A *fistula*, more properly called an *arteriovenous (AV) fistula*, is a surgically made connection between an artery and a vein. Once it is created, it is a natural part of the body. The surgery is usually performed by a vascular surgeon, who specializes in arteries and veins. Generally, a fistula is placed under the skin in the forearm of the *non-dominant arm*—the arm that is used least frequently—but it can be placed in the upper arm if the blood vessels in the forearm are not suitable for a fistula or, in rarer cases, in the leg. Figure 3.1 shows you what a fistula looks like.

When I discuss fistulas with my patients, they commonly ask two questions: "Why is having a fistula created so important?" and "Why does it take so much time before it's ready for use?" Concerning the first question, of all the types of dialysis access, the fistula lasts longest (sometimes decades), is least prone to infection and clotting, and has the greatest *clearance*—which means that it permits the greatest flow of blood during dialysis. The bottom line is that the greater the clearance, the better the dialysis. Remember that the job of dialysis is the filtration of uremic toxins from the body. This filtration depends on good blood flow through the dialysis access, and a well-functioning fistula has very good blood flow—better than that of any other dialysis access.

As to the second question, as already mentioned, the fistula cannot be surgically created and matured in a day. First, after an initial consultation with a vascular surgeon, the surgeon will likely schedule a procedure called *vein mapping*. This is a special ultrasound test that can evaluate how suitable the veins close to the surface of the skin are for placement of an access. If the vessels are found to be adequate, a procedure is scheduled by the vascular surgeon to create the fistula. Performed in the hospital, placement of a fistula is usually same-day surgery, which means that no overnight stay is needed.

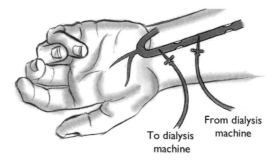

From dialysis machine

To dialysis machine

Figure 3.1. The Hemodialysis Fistula.
This access is a surgically created direct connection between an artery and a vein. Two needles are inserted into the fistula—one to withdraw blood from the body, and one to return the filtered blood to the body.

Once the surgery has been completed, the fistula has to mature and develop. You see, connecting an artery to a vein causes more blood flow to the vein. This makes the vein grow larger and stronger, which means that it's easier to insert needles during repeated dialysis. For many people, the fistula matures in an average of two months. For some people, though, especially if they have diabetes mellitus (DM) or peripheral vascular disease (PVD)—two conditions that often coexist—the fistula needs more time. After the surgery, you may be instructed to perform certain hand exercises, such as squeezing a ball, to help the fistula develop. The vascular surgeon will see you in follow-up and will usually have the final say as to when the access is ready for use.

Unfortunately, not everyone is a candidate for a fistula. Due to small blood vessels and health disorders such as those mentioned above, it is sometimes difficult to create this type of access. Even if one is successfully placed and developed, problems sometimes arise down the line. For instance, *stenosis,* which is an abnormal narrowing of the vein or artery, can lead to decreased blood flow or clotting. In such a case, a graft is the next best option.

Care of the Non-Dominant Arm

If you have not yet had a dialysis access created, your doctor may have instructed you to "save your arm for dialysis." Preferably, you will be asked to save your non-dominant arm—the one that you use the least. (If you write with your right hand, your left arm is non-dominant, and vice versa.). Your job, then, is to do what you can to maintain the integrity, or soundness, of your arm so that the blood vessels will be as healthy as possible when it comes time to create an access. This means that your arm should not be used to measure blood pressure, to draw blood, or for the placement of intravenous lines if you happen to be in the hospital.

When a blood pressure reading is taken, the blood vessels are "squeezed." Over time, this can affect the integrity of the vessels. The needles used to puncture vessels for blood draws and IV access can cause trauma and inflammation to that area. Think about the number of blood draws you have over a period of months or years. If you happen to be a "hard stick"—in other words, if it's sometimes difficult to "find" a vein for a blood test—you may need multiple "tries" over different areas. Over time, these micro-traumas to the vessels lead to scar formation, which can make it difficult to create a good, long-lasting access.

If your dialysis access has already been created, no one should ever take a blood pressure on that arm or use it for blood draws or IVs. As you will read in the next chapter, blood draws are routinely obtained once a month on dialysis. When a test needs to be performed, see if the blood can be drawn on a day when you are on dialysis. The nurse or tech can then access the "dialysis circuit" during treatment, which will help you avoid any unnecessary "sticks" and any resulting injury to the arm.

Remember: No blood pressure, blood draws, or IVs in the non-dominant arm!

The Hemodialysis Graft

As you've already learned, when a vascular surgeon evaluates blood vessels for a dialysis access, he sometimes finds that the vessels are not large and healthy enough to support a fistula. Alternatively, a fistula may be created but either fail to mature or develop problems after repeated use. In these cases, a graft can be used instead.

Unlike a fistula, which directly connects an artery to a vein, a *graft* is created through the indirect connection of an artery to a vein through a synthetic tube that allows the blood to flow from one blood vessel to another. (See Figure 3.2.) Like a fistula, a graft is usually placed under the skin of the forearm of the non-dominant arm, although if the blood vessels in the forearm aren't in good condition, it can be placed in the upper arm or the leg. The placement of a graft usually requires an overnight hospital stay so that you can be observed after surgery. The time it takes for a graft to mature is much shorter than that for a fistula— usually, about two weeks instead of two months.

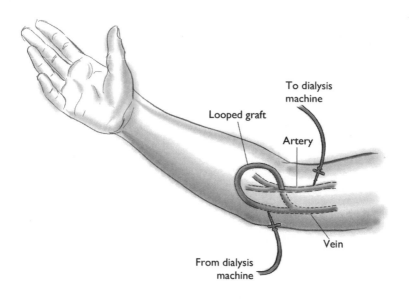

Figure 3.2. The Hemodialysis Graft.
This access is a surgically created indirect connection between an artery and a vein through a synthetic tube that attaches the two blood vessels. Two needles are inserted in the graft—one to withdraw blood from the body, and one to return the filtered blood to the body.

Although a graft is sometimes the best access available for a patient, it is not without potential problems. Compared with a fistula, it has a higher risk of infection and blood clotting. Also, it usually doesn't last as long as a fistula. Although dialysis clearance (blood flow) is good with a graft, it is not as good as that of a fistula.

The Hemodialysis Catheter

A *hemodialysis catheter* is a small, flexible tube that is inserted in a vein to allow blood to flow in and out of your body. (See Figure 3.3.) This is a relatively temporary access that is placed in the neck, chest, or leg when a person needs emergency dialysis in a hospital, when dialysis has to begin before a fistula or graft is able to mature, or when a graft or fistula fails during the course of dialysis.

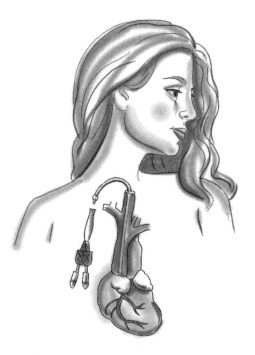

Figure 3.3. The Hemodialysis Catheter.
This access is a flexible tube that is inserted in a vein—in this case, the jugular vein in the neck—to allow blood to flow in and out of the body. The catheter extends outside of the body, where two chambers allow a two-way flow of blood—one, from the body to the dialysis machine, and the other, from the machine to the bloodstream.

There are two types of dialysis catheters. A *temporary dialysis catheter* is one that can be used only in the hospital, usually in the case of an emergency. It is placed in either the subclavian vein or the internal jugular vein in the neck, or, in extreme emergencies, in the femoral vein in the groin area. A *permanent dialysis catheter* permits you to go home with the tube still in place. In this case, a large vein—most commonly, the jugular vein in the neck—is accessed and the tube is "tunneled" under the skin, usually under the collarbone, to increase comfort and minimize complications. Please understand that in this case, the word "permanent" does not mean "forever." These tunneled dialysis catheters often last for several months, but they do not permit good blood flow, are more prone to infection than fistulas and grafts, and can cause narrowing of the vein in which they are placed. They are considered a bridge to a longer-lasting dialysis access, such as a graft or, preferably, a fistula.

Understanding How a Hemodialysis Access Is Used

Now that you know a little about each of the three types of hemodialysis access, you might be wondering how each access is used during the dialysis process. If you have a mature fistula or graft, two needles are inserted through the skin into the access—one for withdrawing blood from the body, and the other for returning the filtered blood to the body. These needles are fairly large in order to accommodate the volume of blood that moves from your body to the dialysis machine, and from the machine back to you. Healthcare professionals operating in dialysis centers usually rotate sites so that the needles are not inserted in the same place during every session. This allows the puncture sites to heal and prevents weakening of any one area. If you have chosen home HD, you may be trained to use the *buttonhole technique,* in which a tunnel of scar tissue is created under your skin to make the insertion of dialysis needles easier and more comfortable. (Think of putting an earring through a pierced ear.)

When a catheter is used in HD, no needles are necessary because the catheter extends outside the body. A catheter has two chambers to allow a two-way flow of blood. One chamber is used to move the blood from the body to the dialysis machine; the other, to move the blood from the machine back to the bloodstream.

ACCESS FOR PERITONEAL DIALYSIS

If you have chosen peritoneal dialysis, or PD, your access will be very different from that of a hemodialysis patient. In your case, a surgeon will insert a catheter through the abdominal wall and into the abdominal (peritoneal) cavity. A portion of the catheter will extend outside your body, near your navel, providing a way to attach the bags of the dialysis fluid, or dialysate. (See Figure 3.4.) The catheter is sealed between uses.

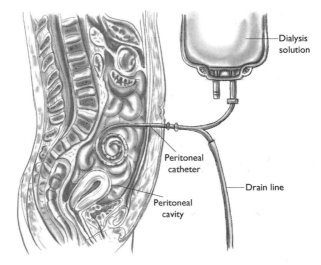

Figure 3.4. The Peritoneal Dialysis Catheter.
The peritoneal dialysis catheter is inserted through the abdominal wall, into the abdominal cavity. The fresh dialysis solution flows from a bag into the peritoneal cavity. After a "dwell time," the solution is removed through a drain tube, into an empty bag.

The permanent PD access is generally created as an outpatient procedure, usually with local anesthesia and an intravenous sedative. A sterile dressing will remain in place for about a week, and will probably be changed by your PD nurse during dialysis training sessions. The healing time takes from two to three weeks, after which, the access can be used for dialysis. Generally, the access lasts for several years, and can be used for both continuous ambulatory peritoneal dialysis (CAPD) and automated peritoneal dialysis (APD). This means that if, like many people, you start off with the manual form of PD and you later transition to the automated form, you will not have to get a different catheter.

In the discussion of accesses for hemodialysis, we talked about the clearance (blood flow) for each type of access. How does a peritoneal catheter measure up? PD is very different from HD, and the clearance actually depends on how well the membrane in your abdominal cavity works as a filter. As mentioned in the previous chapter, *residual kidney function*—any remaining ability of your kidneys to filter wastes from your blood—is important and will affect your peritoneal dialysis prescription. That being said, PD does a very good job of filtering the blood.

Any catheter, including a PD catheter, tends to be more prone to infection than a fistula or graft simply because it protrudes from the body. While there is some risk of *peritonitis (per-a-toe-night-is)*—inflammation of the peritoneum, usually caused by bacterial infection—proper use and care of the catheter can minimize this risk. That's why you usually need a couple of weeks of training in PD and why diligent care of the PD access is so important. (See page 46.)

Understanding How a Peritoneal Access Is Used

Because a PD catheter extends from the body, no needles are involved, and using the access is relatively easy. If you are using ambulatory peritoneal dialysis, the bag of dialysate fluid is attached to the catheter by means of the plastic tubing that comes with the bag. This tubing is detached once the peritoneal cavity is filled with fluid. After the several-hour dwelling period in which the dialysate is allowed to sit in the cavity, an empty bag is attached to the catheter and the fluid is drained out.

Do You Need a Fistula if You're Using Peritoneal Dialysis?

If you are using or considering the use of PD, you probably think that you don't need a fistula, which is a type of access employed in hemodialysis (see page 36). But I recommend that everyone, regardless of their chosen dialysis mode, have a fistula created if at all possible. Then, if something happens to the access you normally use, you will have a backup that will enable you to have hemodialysis without the inconvenient use of HD catheters.

If you are using automated PD, the catheter is attached to a machine called a cycler, which controls the timing of the exchanges, including the filling of the peritoneal cavity with clean solution and the draining of the used solution.

CARE OF YOUR DIALYSIS ACCESS

Because dialysis is a long-term lifesaving therapy, and because its success is so dependent on your access, it's important to take proper care of your access, to be aware of signs that your access is in good shape, and—more important—to be alert to signs of clotting, infection, or other problems. Don't rely solely on your healthcare team to make sure that your access is healthy. Although a member of your team should be contacted whenever you note something unusual, remember that you are probably the only one who will be able to check your access on a daily basis. The following recommendations should help you keep your lifeline healthy and functioning.

Care of a Fistula or Graft

• Wash the skin over your access daily, and especially before a dialysis treatment.

• If you have dialysis in a dedicated facility, ask a member of your healthcare team what the proper protocol is for preparing your skin before needles are placed in your access. Then make sure that these techniques are used before every session.

• At the beginning and end of every dialysis treatment, make sure that both you and the staff are wearing surgical masks that cover the nose and mouth. You don't need to wear a mask during the treatment, but by making sure that everyone is using one when you're being attached to and detached from the dialysis machine, you will decrease the risk of infection.

• Learn how to hold patches against your access after the dialysis needles are removed and in case the site bleeds after treatment. If you have dialysis in a facility, it's a good idea to keep an emergency supply of gauze dressings with you so that you'll be able to stop any bleeding that occurs on the way home.

• Every day, whether or not you're having dialysis, place the middle of your hand over your access and check for a *thrill*—a vibration or pulse indicating that blood is flowing through your access. If you don't feel the thrill, call your doctor right away. He can use a stethoscope to listen to your access for a *bruit (brew-ee)*, a whooshing sound. If there is neither a thrill nor a bruit, it can mean that there is a blood clot in the access and that you need to be "declotted" by an interventional radiologist and/or a vascular surgeon as soon as possible.

• Watch the skin over the access for signs of infection—redness, tenderness, or pus. Report these signs as soon as possible to your nurse or doctor.

• Be alert to signs of an *aneurysm*—a bulge in a blood vessel—and notify your nurse or doctor immediately. The access may require surgery or may simply need to be monitored.

• Protect your access arm by not using it to carry heavy items, by not wearing tight-fitting clothes, and by not sleeping on it. (For more information on protecting your arm, see the inset on page 38.)

Care of a Hemodialysis Catheter

• Be sure to keep your catheter dressing clean and dry. Always wash and dry your hands and put on a surgical mask before handling the site.

• Make sure that your dialysis team cleans the area before dialysis and changes the dressing at the end of each session.

• *Never* remove the cap at the end of the catheter. Only the dialysis team should open the catheter. Make sure that the clamps remain closed, as well. If a cap comes off, contact your dialysis team immediately.

• If any part of the catheter develops a leak or hole, ensure that the tube is clamped off above the hole. Then contact your dialysis nurse or doctor right away.

- When taking a shower, use a special plastic covering to tightly seal your access. If moisture gets in, it will increase the risk of infection.

- Every day, check the *exit site*—the area where the catheter and skin surface make contact. If you see redness, swelling, or any discharge, or if you feel any pain when you touch the site, call your dialysis nurse or doctor immediately. This can indicate infection and requires prompt attention. Ask your team about other symptoms that should be reported.

Care of a Peritoneal Catheter

- Be sure to keep your catheter dressing clean and dry. Every time you handle the site—at the start or end of a treatment or after taking a shower, for instance—put on a surgical mask and wash and dry your hands. After a treatment and after each shower, clean and dry the site before applying a fresh dressing according to your doctor's instructions. To reduce the risk of infection, he will probably instruct you to put a pea-sized amount of an antibiotic cream such as gentamicin in the center of the dressing.

- When taking a shower, use a special plastic covering to tightly seal your access. If moisture gets in, it will increase the risk of infection.

- Never apply any cream or other substance to your exit site without getting an okay from your doctor or nurse.

- If you see that a small scab has formed at the exit site, do not pick at or remove it. Just allow it to heal.

- To prevent tension and tugging on the catheter, always keep it secured to your skin with a piece of tape near the exit site. Avoid wearing clothes that will irritate the site through rubbing or pressure.

- Regularly examine your catheter for cracks. Cracks can allow bacteria to enter and cause infection.

- Be alert to any changes in the fluid that's drained from the abdominal cavity during an exchange. Cloudy fluid may indicate peritonitis. This should immediately be brought to the attention of your doctor or dialysis nurse so that it can be treated with antibiotics.

• Every day, check the *exit site*—the area where the catheter and skin surface make contact. If you see redness, swelling, or any discharge, or if you feel any pain when you touch the site, call your dialysis nurse or doctor immediately. This can indicate infection and requires prompt attention. Ask your dialysis team about other symptoms that should be reported.

IN CONCLUSION

The importance of your dialysis access cannot be overstated. It truly is your lifeline. Understanding what your access is, how it is used during dialysis, and how you can keep it healthy and troubleshoot any problems is vital to dialysis success. If you have chosen home dialysis, you will have most of the responsibility for taking care of your access and heading off any problems. But even if you have your treatments in a dialysis center, you should make sure that your healthcare team uses the proper protocol, and on those days when you don't have treatments, you should protect your access and be on the alert for signs of infection and clotting.

In the next chapter, you will discover another way to take an active role in your health as your learn the value of monthly blood work.

4

$\mathcal{R}$eviewing Your Monthly Blood Work

During every month of your dialysis, on the first or the second week, blood work is obtained for review by your doctor, nurse, and dietitian. These tests are crucial because they not only define how well your dialysis is removing toxins from your blood, but also provide markers of your total body health, including the condition of your blood and bones, the soundness of your diet, and the presence of inflammation. It is a common practice for dialysis units to give you a copy of your monthly blood work with explanations of what can be improved through medication, nutrition, or a change in your dialysis treatment. This chapter will help you better understand your lab results by providing a discussion of each test that is commonly ordered on a monthly basis. You will begin by learning about the tests that show blood health and move on to those that help your team evaluate your bones, nutrition and inflammation, and dialysis clearance. You will also learn about a key nutrient that helps maintain normal heart function. Although the focus is on monthly blood tests, I will also discuss some important tests that may be performed less frequently. The inset on page 50 provides an at-a-glance look at all of these tests and their goal values.

Depending on your dialysis center and any other medical conditions you may have, tests other than those discussed in this chapter—a cholesterol panel and a blood glucose level, for instance—may be ordered by your doctor. This chapter focuses on the most common tests that are ordered by nephrologists for their dialysis patients.

An At-a-Glance Look at Common Blood Tests

This chapter helps you understand those blood tests that you will have on a monthly basis throughout your dialysis treatment, as well as a few tests that will be performed less frequently but are still of vital importance. The table below gives you an at-a-glance view of all these tests, how often they're done, and what the healthy treatment range is. Be aware that in some cases, the treatment range depends on the type of dialysis with which you're being treated, so it's important to note the third column, "Type of Dialysis." Because everyone is unique, it's also essential to ask your nephrologist if all of the target levels stated below are right for you, or if in some instances, your goal is different.

Common Blood Work Tests and Healthy Treatment Ranges

Test	When It's Performed	Type of Dialysis	Healthy Treatment Range
Tests for Blood Health			
Hemoglobin (Hgb)	Once a month	All types	10–12 g/dL
Hematocrit (Hct)	Once a month	All types	30–36 percent
White Blood Cell Count (WBC)	Once a month	All types	4,500–10,500 cells per mcL
Platelets (plts)	Once a month	All types	150,000–450,000 cells per mcL
Iron Saturation Level	Every 3 months	All types	20 percent or greater
Ferritin	Every 3 months	All types of hemodialysis	200 ng/mL or greater
	Every 3 months	Peritoneal dialysis	100 ng/mL or greater
Tests for Bone Health			
Phosphorus	Once a month	All types	3.5–5.5 mg/dL
Calcium	Once a month	All types	8.4–9.5 mg/dL
Parathyroid Hormone (PTH)	Every 3 months	All types	150–600 pg/mL
Magnesium	As requested by your doctor	All types	1.6–2.6 mg/dL

Test	When It's Performed	Type of Dialysis	Healthy Treatment Range
Tests of Nutritional Status and Inflammation			
Albumin	Once a month	All types of hemodialysis	4.0 mg/dL
	Once a month	Peritoneal dialysis	3.5 mg/dL
Ferritin	Every 3 months	All types of hemodialysis	200 ng/mL or greater
	Every 3 months	Peritoneal dialysis	100 ng/mL or greater
Test for Heart Health			
Potassium	Once a month	All types	3.5–5.0 mEq/L
Tests of Toxin Clearance			
Urea Reduction Ratio	Once a month	Standard in-center hemodialysis	65 percent or greater per treatment
	Once a month	Nocturnal in-center hemodialysis	65 percent or greater per treatment
	Once a month	Home hemodialysis	35–40 percent or greater per treatment
	About every 3 months	Peritoneal dialysis	65 percent or greater per treatment
Kt/V	Once a month	Standard in-center hemodialysis	1.2 or greater per treatment
	Once a month	Nocturnal in-center hemodialysis	1.2 or greater per treatment
	Once a month	Home hemodialysis	.5–.6 per treatment
	About every 3 months	Continuous ambulatory peritoneal dialysis	2.0 per week
		Automated peritoneal dialysis	2.1 per week

BLOOD WORK RELATED TO YOUR BLOOD HEALTH

In Chapter 1, you learned one reason why kidney disease can lead to *anemia,* an abnormally low level of red blood cells. In actuality, there are a number of ways in which both advanced kidney disease and dialysis itself can result in or contribute to this condition:

- Kidneys that have failed are not able to make the hormone *erythropoietin,* which normally stimulates the bone marrow to produce red blood cells.

- The accumulation of uremic toxins may depress bone marrow function.

- Iron deficiency, caused by dialyzer-related blood loss and frequent blood sampling, can contribute to anemia.

- Folate, vitamin B_{12}, and other B vitamins important to red blood cell production can be lost through dialysis.

- In advanced kidney disease, the lifespan of red blood cells can be shorter than the normal lifespan of three months.

- Platelets, the components of blood that aid in blood clotting, usually don't work well in the presence of uremia, making bleeding—and, therefore, anemia—more common.

- The inflammation associated with kidney disease can affect the body's ability to produce red blood cells.

On dialysis, the monthly lab tests that are associated with blood work include a *complete blood count* and *iron studies.* It should be noted that the blood sample is usually collected at the very beginning of the dialysis session, as the dialysis process can cause false counts.

The Complete Blood Count

The complete blood count, or CBC, is a measure of many factors. However, your doctor is most concerned with the following four components: the *hemoglobin (heme-moe-glow-bin);* the *hematocrit (he-matto-krit); the white blood cell count;* and the *platelets (play-tell-ets).*

Since *hemoglobin (Hgb)* is the protein in red blood cells that carries oxygen to tissues, and the *hematocrit (Hct)* shows the percentage of blood composed of red blood cells, these two tests let you know if anemia is present. For someone on dialysis, the optimal hemoglobin level is somewhere between 10 and 12 g/dL (grams per deciliter), and a healthy hematocrit is 30 to 36 percent. In Chapter 5, you'll learn about the medications that can be used to boost labs to these goal levels. (To learn more about the goal hemoglobin level, see the inset on page 55.)

White blood cells (WBCs)—also known as *leukocytes*—are an important part of the body's defense system. They kill bacteria, combat disease, fight allergic reactions, and destroy old and damaged cells. The normal range for anyone, including a dialysis patient, is 4,500 to 10,500 cells per mcL (microliter). When the WBC count is elevated—in other words, higher than 10,500 per mcL—it may indicate a physical trauma or infection, with infection being the greatest concern to your physician. However, a WBC count that's *lower* than 4,500 can also be a sign of certain infections, such as viral illnesses. If blood is drawn in the middle of a dialysis session, there can be a falsely low reading.

Platelets (plts), also called *thrombocytes*, have as their chief function the clotting of blood. A normal platelet count is between 150,000 and 450,000 cells per mcL (microliter). A platelet count above 450,000 can indicate infection, inflammation, or an iron deficiency. A platelet count below 150,000 can be caused by a reaction to a medication. For instance, heparin, which is a common blood thinner used during dialysis to prevent blood clotting, can lower the platelet count in some people.

Iron Studies

In addition to the monthly blood count tests, every three months, iron studies are collected. These labs, which include an *iron saturation level* and a *ferritin level*, are performed because there must be an adequate amount of iron stores in order for erythropoietin-stimulating agents (ESAs) such as Epogen to work.

The *iron saturation level* indicates how much iron is circulating in the blood. Nephrologists generally shoot for 20 percent or greater. The *ferritin level* represents how much iron is stored in the body. An adequate ferritin level is 200 ng/mL (nanograms per milliliter) for someone on hemodialysis and 100 ng/mL for someone on peritoneal dialysis. Your nephrologist will look at both the iron saturation and the ferritin levels to determine if you need supplementation with iron. However, a higher-than-normal level of ferritin can indicate inflammation. Because inflammation can prevent iron from being well utilized by the body, iron is not always prescribed in the case of high ferritin levels.

BLOOD WORK RELATED TO YOUR BONE HEALTH

Bone health depends on a complex interplay between the minerals phosphorus and calcium, vitamin D, and a hormone known as parathyroid hormone, or PTH. Healthy kidneys help protect the bones by controlling the body's levels of phosphorus and calcium, and by transforming and activating the vitamin D obtained from sun exposure and diet. Healthy kidneys also play a part in regulating magnesium, another mineral that is important to bone health. As the kidneys fail, the amounts of all of these substances get out of kilter, and the bones suffer.

Your monthly blood work monitors your bone health by determining your levels of phosphorus, calcium, and parathyroid hormone. Many dialysis centers, on request, will test for magnesium and vitamin D, as well, but these substances may not be part of routine blood testing. As you learn about each of the substances discussed below, keep in mind that abnormalities in these values affect not just your bone health, but also the condition of your heart and blood vessels.

Phosphorus Levels

When a person with normal kidney function eats a meal that's high in phosphorus, the kidneys eliminate the extra phosphorus through the urine. In advanced kidney disease, the kidneys are unable to remove the mineral, and the level rises. The body, in an effort to restore balance, then changes the levels of vitamin D and parathyroid hormone (PTH), and also leaches calcium out of the bones, weakening the bones and leading to dangerous calcium deposits in the blood vessels and other organs. Very high phosphorus levels can also lead to *pruritis,* the chronic itching mentioned in Chapter 1 (see page 10).

What Is the Goal Hemoglobin Level?

It has taken several years of research to identify a goal hemoglobin, or Hgb, level. Years ago, it was recognized that an Hgb of 8 g/dL or lower increased the risk of death by adding to the workload of the heart. Remember that hemoglobin is the oxygen-bearing component of blood, and the heart pumps blood to the rest of the body as a means of delivering this oxygen to the organs and tissues. The lower the Hgb level, the more blood is needed to deliver the necessary oxygen, and the harder the heart must work to keep the organs supplied. Over time, the added stress can result in *left ventricular hypertrophy,* or LVH, a thickening of the muscle of the heart's left ventricle. LVH is a risk factor for sudden cardiac death.

Once the association was made between low Hgb and heart disease, it was decided that a higher Hgb must be better. But several studies showed that maintaining an Hgb level greater than 13 g/dL is actually connected with a shorter lifespan. The current goal is to keep the Hgb level between 10 and 12 g/dL, and, when needed, to use erythropoietin-stimulating drugs to raise Hgb to a healthy level.

In monthly blood work, a healthy phosphorus level for a patient on any type of dialysis is between 3.5 and 5.5 mg/dL (milligrams per deciliter). The control of these levels is very difficult for people with kidney disease, however. Standard in-center dialysis removes up to 70 percent of excess phosphorus; in other words, it does not remove all. Because nocturnal and home HD provide more treatment time, they eliminate more. One day of peritoneal dialysis removes less phosphorus than standard HD, but treatments are performed on a daily basis. The bottom line is that—regardless of the type of dialysis treatment you're receiving—you will probably be given medications called phosphorus binders if your levels exceed the acceptable range. (You'll learn more about phosphorus binders in the next chapter.) In such a case, most likely, you will also be counseled by a dietitian to avoid foods and beverages that are high in phosphorus. (See page 129 of Chapter 9 for specific dietary information.)

Calcium Levels

As you read above, there is a close interplay between calcium and phosphorus. For someone on dialysis, a normal calcium level is between 8.4 and 9.5 mg/dL (milligrams per deciliter). The goal of your nephrologist is to keep your calcium within that range to help protect the health of your bones. If your level is on the lower side, she may recommend calcium replacement. If your levels are on the higher side, your physician will probably not suggest calcium supplements.

Parathyroid Hormone (PTH) Levels

Produced by the parathyroid gland, the parathyroid hormone has as its chief function the control of the blood level of calcium. As mentioned earlier, the interplay between PTH and certain nutrients is complex, but put simply, high phosphorus levels lead to high PTH levels, resulting in a condition known as *secondary hyperparathyroidism (hyper-para-thigh-roid-ism)*. This condition can result in a weakening of bones and the calcification of tissues and organs, including the lungs, heart, blood vessels, joints, and skin.

Although a normal level of PTH is between 150 and 600 pg/mL (picograms per milliliter), many doctors aim for the lower end of the range. Vitamin D can keep PTH levels on an even keel, but healthy kidneys are needed to turn vitamin D into its active form. For that reason, when high PTH is a problem, physicians often prescribe activated vitamin D to suppress parathyroid hormone production. Hemodialysis patients are given a prescription intravenous form of this medication during dialysis, while those using peritoneal dialysis are prescribed an oral form of activated vitamin D. (You'll learn more about activated vitamin D on page 70 of the next chapter.) Parathyroid hormones are then checked regularly to make sure that PTH is being adequately suppressed but not over-suppressed.

Magnesium

Magnesium plays a role in hundreds of the body's biochemical reactions, and one of its many functions is to protect bone health. But while it is an important mineral, it must be kept in balance. Just as healthy kidneys eliminate excess phorphorus from the body, they also filter out any excess magnesium. As you might expect, in someone with kidney failure, magnesium can reach unhealthy levels. Yet, this is not always the case. Because of poor eating and malnourishment, some people on dialysis actually have lower-than-normal levels of this mineral.

Magnesium is not part of a standard monthly blood test for dialysis patients, but it can be tested at the physician's discretion. Generally, a normal range is considered to be between 1.6 and 2.6 mg/dL (milligrams per deciliter). When doctors find that the level is low, magnesium supplementation and a nutritional evaluation may be ordered. When magnesium levels are found to be high, your doctor will most likely review your diet and your medications. Some common over-the-counter medications that may have to be eliminated are Mylanta and Milk of Magnesia, both of which are high in magnesium.

BLOOD WORK RELATED TO NUTRITION AND INFLAMMATION

You may be wondering why nutrition and inflammation are being covered in the same discussion. This is because one of the most important tests in the blood panel—the albumin test—can actually provide information about both nutritional status and infection. This section will first look at albumin and then revisit an important marker that you learned about earlier: ferritin.

Albumin Levels

Albumin is a protein made by the liver. When an individual does not eat enough calories or protein, the liver doesn't have enough protein to make albumin, and blood levels of this protein drop. This is common in dialysis patients, as they often experience a loss of appetite, especially on dialysis days. A normal albumin level is 4.0 mg/dL (milligrams per deciliter) for patients on hemodialysis, and 3.5 mg/dL for patients on peritoneal dialysis. This difference is due to the fact that dialysis treatments filter some protein from the blood along with toxins and waste, and PD does a more thorough job of filtering than HD.

Research has shown that over time, low albumin levels have an adverse effect on lifespan.

Albumin is also important because it is a marker of total body inflammation, and, as you may remember from Chapter 1, chronic kidney disease is a state of inflammation that can affect the entire body. One of my patients generally had an albumin level of 4.0 mg/dL, which is an acceptable level. One month, his level dropped to 3.2 mg/dL. He felt well, and at first, no source of inflammation could be identified. On subsequent evaluation, though, he was found to have a periodontal infection. When the infection was successfully treated, his albumin level improved.

When a low albumin level is found, your nephrologist and nutritionist will probably question you about your diet and possibly ask you to keep a food diary of what you are eating. As a result, they may make dietary recommendations and a modification of your supplement program. Your nephrologist may also look for signs of infection. In some cases, a test for *prealbumin* may be ordered. Like a low albumin level, a low prealbumin level can indicate not only low nourishment but also inflammation. A normal prealbumin level is approximately 20 to 40 mg/dL. When malnutrition and inflammation are both present, the prealbumin level can drop rapidly.

A Second Look at Ferritin

If you recall from the section on blood health, ferritin is a measure of how much iron is stored in your body. Guess what? Ferritin, like albumin, is also a marker of total body inflammation. It is an example of an *acute phase reactant*, which is a substance that increases in response to an acute condition such as infection. When someone is on any form of hemodialysis, an acceptable level of ferritin is 200 ng/mL (nanograms per milliliter). When a patient is on peritoneal dialysis, a healthy level is 100 ng/mL. When inflammation is present, ferritin levels rise. In general levels above 500 ng/mL are associated with moderate inflammation, and levels greater than 1,000 ng/mL indicate a more severe infection or inflammatory condition.

When looking at markers like ferritin and albumin, keep in mind that trends over time are important. Your body is an amazing creation geared to maintain balance and harmony. When albumin levels get progressively lower and ferritin levels rise, your body is providing clues that can help your medical team better address your health problems.

BLOOD WORK RELATED TO YOUR HEART

Earlier in the chapter, I mentioned that in addition to playing a role in bone health, the minerals phosphorus, calcium, and magnesium also affect the condition of your heart. (See page 54.) We've already discussed the healthy levels for these minerals. Now we're going to look at another mineral that's important to heart health—potassium.

Potassium is a vital nutrient because it controls the beat of the heart, as well as performing other functions in the body. But when the kidneys do not function normally and are unable to eliminate excess potassium, levels of this mineral can actually get too high. That's why physicians monitor every dialysis patient's magnesium level. A normal range for potassium is 3.5 to 5 mEq/L (milliequivalents per liter). When potassium levels rise to 6 or 7 mEq/L, your heart can develop an irregular rhythm called an *arrhythmia (a-rith-mee-a)*.

In general, people on peritoneal dialysis have less problems with high potassium than people who are on hemodialysis. Nevertheless, most dialysis diets regulate potassium by limiting high-potassium foods. (You'll learn more about this on page 123 of Chapter 9.)

BLOOD WORK RELATED TO THE CLEARANCE OF TOXINS

A significant question that my patients often ask is, "How well is my dialysis working?" In addition to how you feel, which is an important measure of the treatment's success, there are tests that can objectively answer this question by determining how well the treatment is filtering out a substance called urea from your bloodstream. *Urea* is the toxin that's produced by the body after protein metabolism. Healthy kidneys eliminate urea from the body, but in kidney failure, dialysis has to take over that job. Two tests are used to measure how well dialysis is ridding your body of urea. One is the *urea reduction ratio (URR)* and the other is the *Kt/V*. While many dialysis centers use both tests, the current trend is to focus on the URR as a measure of toxin clearance. Your dialysis team can tell you which tests they use to evaluate the effectiveness of your treatments.

At this point, an important caveat is in order. Goal URR and Kt/V levels have been clearly established only for standard three-times-a-week hemodialysis. It has been more challenging to calculate goal levels for other types of dialysis, and appropriate treatment ranges for home HD, noctural HD, and peritoneal dialysis are still being discussed by dialysis experts. Below, I have tried to give you a general idea of what your numbers are likely to be if you are using one of these treatments, but it is essential to speak to your healthcare team and discuss your particular clearance goals.

The Urea Reduction Ratio (URR)

The URR is performed by taking one blood sample at the beginning of the dialysis session and another at the end of the same session. That way, the dialysis team can get a clear picture of how well the urea is being eliminated from your body. Most dialysis centers collect this information on a monthly basis for all dialysis patients.

The results of the URR are expressed as a percentage of the urea being filtered during your dialysis treatment. When reading your blood work, if you are on three-times-a-week in-center dialysis, you want to see a URR that is at least 65 percent; higher is even better. As I explained earlier, no clear guidelines have been set for the URR for other forms of dialysis. If you are on nocturnal dialysis, the minimum URR is 65 percent, but it is often much higher than this, as the amount of dialysis time is often double that of standard in-center dialysis. The URR for home HD depends on the dialysis prescription provided by your nephrologist. Because home HD involves shorter sessions—each ranges from two and a half to three and a half hours in length—the URR for a single session is generally 35 to 40 percent. If you are on peritoneal dialysis, the URR should be 65 percent or higher. Keep in mind, though, that the Kt/V is the preferred means of evaluating PD effectiveness.

If your dialysis clearance falls below the target number set by your nephrologist, your team may increase the amount of time you spend dialyzing or adjust the machine's rate of flow so that a higher percentage of urea is removed during each session. Another option may be to increase the size of the *dialyzer,* which is the filter found within the dialysis machine. It is the dialyzer that actually cleans your blood when it passes through the machine.

The Kt/V

Like the URR test, the Kt/V usually involves having one blood sample taken before the dialysis treatment and another sample taken at the end of the session. It is often used along with the URR, and if you are on hemodialysis, you will see the two tests listed together on your monthly blood work. When you begin peritoneal dialysis treatments, this test is usually done monthly to make sure that the treatments are adequately filtering the blood. After that, as long as your treatments are going well and your dialysis prescription isn't changed, your doctor will probably check it every three months.

Kt/V is actually a mathematical formula: K refers to clearance (the amount of urea removed by the dialyzer in terms of liters per minute); t is the duration of the treatment in minutes; and V is equivalent to the amount of water in your body. Using these three figures, the computer determines your Kt/V. This calculation takes into account your size, the length of your treatment, your blood flow rate, the amount of urea made by your body during dialysis, and the urea and fluid removed by dialysis.

If you are on three-times-a-week in-center dialysis, your Kt/V should be 1.2 or greater. As is the case with the URR, no strict guidelines have been set for other forms of HD, but the Kt/V for home HD should be around .5 to .6 per treatment, and for nocturnal dialysis, the goal is greater than 1.2 per treatment. In peritoneal dialysis, the weekly goal Kt/V is 2.0 for continuous ambulatory PD, and 2.1 for automated PD. That being said, if a PD patient's Kt/V is 1.7 or greater, her other blood work is acceptable, and she is generally feeling well, her treatments should be seen as providing adequate clearance. In some cases, it can be difficult to raise the Kt/V number despite changes in the dialysis prescription. That's why it's so important to view your blood work as a whole—and to also consider your general well-being—rather than focusing on just one number. Still, for any mode of dialysis, if the Kt/V indicates that the dialysis treatments are not providing adequate filtering of the blood, the dialysis team may recommend changes that will remove more urea.

IN CONCLUSION

You can see how important it is to understand the values provided in your monthly lab reports. When your team hands you a copy of your report, it's vital to read the values, to compare them with those in earlier reports, and to note any trends. Even though you have a healthcare team supporting you, never forget that it is you, the patient, who has the most to gain from keeping on top of your labs. Your active involvement in your own care can make a world of difference in the quality and length of your life.

5

$\mathcal{U}$nderstanding Your Dialysis-Related Medications

A
lthough dialysis takes over some of the essential functions of healthy kidneys, it certainly isn't able to do everything that working kidneys do. It can't stimulate the bone marrow's production of red blood cells; it can't remove all of the toxins that accumulate in the blood; and it can't balance the body's levels of phosphorus, calcium, and parathyroid hormone. In addition, the process of dialysis removes large amounts of important water-soluble vitamins, such as the B-complex vitamins and vitamin C, from your bloodstream, as well as some red blood cells. In some cases, dietary modifications can do a portion of the kidneys' work or make up for the removal of some nutrients through dialysis. (To learn about dietary considerations on dialysis, see Chapter 9.) In the majority of cases, though, medication and supplements are needed to help prevent and/or alleviate kidney- and dialysis-related health problems.

This chapter looks at the most common medications that are provided to dialysis patients to compensate either for the loss of kidney function or for the side effects of the dialysis treatments. (For a quick reference to dialysis-related medications, see Table 5.1 on page 64.) If you want to learn about taking medications for other types of disorders while you're on dialysis, turn to Chapter 7. If you're interested in exploring supplements that can help improve your health and enhance your quality of life, turn to Chapter 8.

MEDICATIONS FOR BLOOD HEALTH

As you learned in previous chapters, the kidneys are responsible for keeping the red blood count high through the production of the bone marrow-stimulating hormone known as *erythropoietin*. When the kidneys no longer function, the result is almost always *anemia*—a lower-

Table 5.1. Common Dialysis-Related Medications

Type of Medication	Examples
Erythropoietin-Stimulating Agents (ESAs)	Epogen (epoetin alfa), Procrit (epoetin alfa), Aranesp (darbepoetin alfa)
Iron Supplements	Venofer (iron sucrose), Ferrlecit (sodium ferric gluconate)
Renal Vitamins	Nephrocaps, Nephroplex
Phosphorus Binders	PhosLo (calcium acetate), Renagel (sevelamer), Renvela (sevelamer carbonate)
Vitamin D Analogues	Zemplar (paricalcitol), Hectorol (doxercalciferol), Rocaltrol (calcitriol)
Calcimimetics	Sensipar (cinacalcet)

than-normal red blood cell count that causes symptoms such as fatigue, dizziness, an irregular heartbeat, shortness of breath, and even cognitive problems. Two types of medications are given to the dialysis patient to prevent serious anemia—erythropoietin-stimulating agents and iron supplements. Each of these mainstays of dialysis medication is discussed on the following pages.

Why It Is Taken	How It Is Taken	Possible Side Effects
Stimulates the bones' production of red blood cells.	Intravenously (during dialysis) or by subcutaneous injection.	Fever, dizziness, nausea, vomiting, diarrhea, hypertension, pain and swelling at the injection site.
Raises the level of iron to fuel the production of red blood cells.	Intravenously (during dialysis or as separate infusion).	Gastrointestinal pain, nausea, breathing problems, rash and other skin problems, chest pain, low blood pressure.
Replaces water-soluble vitamins (like B-complex and C) that are lost during dialysis.	Orally, usually once daily.	Drowsiness, headache, mild diarrhea, nausea.
Prevents a toxic buildup of phosphorus.	Orally, with meals and snacks.	Upset stomach, nausea, vomiting, diarrhea.
Lowers levels of parathyroid hormone (PTH) and increases blood calcium levels.	Intravenously (during dialysis) or orally.	Dizziness, lightheadedness, nausea. More rarely, allergic symptoms such as rash, hives, swelling of lips or tongue, difficulty breathing; chest pain; palpitations.
Mimics calcium to lower levels of parathyroid hormone (PTH).	Orally, once daily, usually with dinner.	Nausea and stomach upset. Rarely, numbness or tightness around mouth, changed heart rate, muscle tightness or contraction, shortness of breath, seizures.

Medications to Raise Red Blood Cell Blood Count

Erythropoietin-stimulating agents, or *ESAs*—also called *recombinant erythropoietin*—are man-made versions of the natural hormone erythropoietin. Like the hormone, these drugs stimulate the bones' production of red blood cells, which are then released by the bone marrow into the bloodstream.

Several different ESAs are used. Epogen and Procrit are two brands of epoetin alfa, and Aranesp is the brand name for darbepoetin alfa. All of these drugs work well, the difference being that Aranesp is a longer-acting medication than the others, and thus has to be taken less frequently. Epogen and Procrit may be given three times a week, while Aranesp may be provided only once a week. The dose is tailored to each patient based on the targeted hemoglobin level, which, as you learned in Chapter 4, is 10 to 12 g/dL. The minimum effective dose is given as a means of reducing side effects. If you have any type of cancer, your nephrologist will speak to your oncologist to determine if ESAs are appropriate for you. In some people with malignancies, the use of these drugs has been associated with tumor growth. Because these drugs can raise blood pressure, they may not be given when someone's blood pressure is high to begin with—for instance, at the beginning of a dialysis session, when fluid gain may cause hypertension. If blood pressure becomes lower during the treatment, the ESA can then be provided. Other possible side effects of these medications include fever, dizziness, nausea and vomiting, diarrhea, and pain and swelling at the site of the injection. Notify your dialysis nurse or physician if you experience any of these symptoms.

If you are on in-center hemodialysis, including nocturnal dialysis, your ESA will be given intravenously as part of the dialysis process. In other words, there will be no additional needle sticks. If you are on home hemodialysis or peritoneal dialysis, you may have to visit the dialysis center for your injections. Alternatively, you may be able to administer your own injections at home. At this point, you may be asking yourself, "Can I really give myself an injection?" Fortunately, these medications can be injected *subcutaneously (sub-q-tane-ee-us-lee),* or under the skin, so they are really easy to administer. They are very similar to the insulin injections that many people who have diabetes routinely give themselves.

Iron Supplements

Iron has to be present in order for the production of red blood cells to take place. No matter how much the bone marrow is "revved up" by the ESAs, without adequate iron, red blood cells will be fewer in number and smaller in size. Trying to make blood cells without iron is like trying to drive a car without gas; no matter how "souped up" the engine is, it's not going to run. Because small amounts of iron are lost during each hemodialysis session through the loss of red blood cells, eventually, most people who are on dialysis need to receive iron in order to fuel blood cell production.

You may now be wondering if you can simply take over-the-counter iron tablets to supplement your body's stores of this mineral. In most cases, oral iron is not sufficient to supply what is needed. Also, many

Treating Anemia with ESAs

Currently, nephrologists strive for a hemoglobin (Hgb) level between 10 and 12 g/dL. (See the inset on page 55.) Your doctor will prescribe an ESA dosage with the goal of keeping your Hgb within that range without the levels *cycling*, or going up and down, like a yo-yo. If your Hgb drops below this range, he will increase the dosage. If it rises above 12, he may decrease the dosage or even stop the medication for a while. However, there is a danger that if the medication is stopped completely, the Hgb will drop too much after a few weeks. By monitoring your monthly blood work and noting trends, your doctor will learn how much he can lessen or increase your ESA dose to avoid your Hgb from going above or below the desired range.

Sometimes, regardless of the amounts of ESA and iron you receive, you can still be anemic. If your labs show that your iron stores are adequate, your doctor will begin looking for any nutritional deficiencies, such as deficiencies in B_{12} or folic acid, that might be contributing to the anemia. He will also look for signs of infection or inflammation, as these are other possible causes of low red blood cell counts. These days, through careful iron management and the use of ESAs, most dialysis patients are able to experience the good energy levels that result from having a healthy red blood cell count.

people find that these pills upset their stomach and cause constipation. Nephrologists usually advise against taking oral iron because the intravenous form is given during treatments. If you nevertheless decide to use oral iron, take it at least an hour before or after your other medications so that it can be better absorbed and does not interfere with the absorption of your other meds. Take some vitamin C along with the iron, as even small amounts, like 250 mg, can increase the body's absorption of oral iron. But please understand that even if you take iron tablets, you will also likely be prescribed intravenous iron, because the amount of the mineral provided by the tablets will not be sufficient to raise your red blood cell count.

Common intravenous iron formulations include Venofer (iron sucrose) and Ferrlecit (sodium ferric gluconate). If you are an in-center HD patient, you can receive these supplements during your dialysis treatment. If you are doing home HD or PD, you may be asked to come into the dialysis center—monthly or more frequently, as needed—to have an intravenous infusion of iron, which usually lasts for only one or two hours. Side effects of intravenous iron are generally minimal, but may include gastrointestinal pains, nausea, breathing problems, rash and other skin problems, chest pain, and low blood pressure. Any severe or persistent symptoms should be reported to your physician.

"KIDNEY" VITAMINS

The dialysis process itself—especially hemodialysis—can rob your body of water-soluble nutrients such as the B-complex vitamins and vitamin C. Although a good diet can help replace the lost nutrients, the problem is that many dialysis patients have a poor appetite. That's why most nephrologists suggest daily "kidney" vitamin pills, called *renal vitamins*. These generally contain the B vitamins, and often vitamin C and zinc, as well. Nephrocaps and Nephroplex are just two of the brands that may be prescribed.

Normally, side effects are rare with renal vitamins, but these supplements can cause drowsiness, headache, mild diarrhea, or nausea. Call your doctor if these symptoms become bothersome or if you experience more severe side effects such as numbness or tingling of the skin; or allergic reactions such as rash, hives, or difficulty breathing.

Why can't you just take a standard multivitamin? A multivitamin pill often doesn't supply enough of the nutrients you need. Even worse, it provides nutrients that you not only don't require, but shouldn't take while you're on dialysis. For instance, most multivitamins contain vitamin A, a fat-soluble vitamin that can build up to toxic levels in a person with kidney failure. If you are already taking a multivitamin, be sure to review the formula with your doctor or dietitian to see if it should be discontinued.

Your renal vitamins should be taken at the same time every day. Most people take them either first thing in the morning or late at night. They do not have to be accompanied with a meal.

MEDICATIONS FOR BONE HEALTH

Because your kidneys are no longer able to remove excess phosphorus from your blood, this mineral can accumulate to unhealthy levels in your blood. This, in turn, will cause changes in the blood levels of calcium and parathyroid hormone (PTH)—all of which, if left unchecked, is bad for your bones. To maintain your bone health, your nephrologist will prescribe medications that lower both phosphorus and PTH.

Medications That Lower Phosphorus

In addition to counseling you to maintain a low-phosphorous diet, your doctor may prescribe a type of medication called a *phosphorus binder* or *phosphate binder*. These medications are prescribed for anyone—on any form of dialysis—who has a phosphorus level greater than 5 mg/dL. If your level of this mineral is lower, you may not need to take a phosphorus binder, or you may need only a low dosage.

Phosphorus binders work in the intestinal tract by binding to the phosphorus found in foods and causing the mineral to be eliminated from the body rather than absorbed into the blood. This category of medication includes calcium-containing binders, like PhosLo (calcium acetate), and binders that contain no calcium, such as Renagel (sevelamer) and Renvela (sevelamer carbonate). There are also liquid formulations for people who have trouble swallowing the many pills often needed on hemodialysis.

Depending on your blood work, you may be told to take from one to three pills—or the equivalent in liquid—at each meal. Be careful to follow your doctor's advice to the letter about the timing of the dosage. Some phosphorus binders should be taken just before eating, but others should be taken during or immediately after a meal because dosing on an empty stomach can cause nausea and vomiting. Since the binders can interfere with the body's absorption of iron supplements as well as antibiotics, digoxin, and anti-seizure medications, take these other drugs at least one hour before or three hours after your binders. If you forget to take your binder with a meal, try to take it within thirty minutes of eating. If this is not possible, just skip the dose. Do *not* double your next dose.

The most common side effects of phosphorus binders—both calcium-based and non-calcium-based formulations—are stomach upset, nausea, vomiting, and diarrhea. Call your doctor if these problems become severe, and seek immediate medical attention if you have symptoms of an allergic reaction such as rash, swelling of the tongue or throat, trouble breathing, or dizziness.

Medications That Lower PTH

High levels of PTH can cause loss of bone calcium and phosphorus, as well as inflammation of the bones, muscles, and tendons. Two basic types of medication are used to treat *hyperparathyroidism,* or an excessive production of the parathyroid hormone. They are *activated vitamin D* and *calcimimetics (cal-see-mim-ettiks).*

Activated vitamin D, sometimes referred to as a *vitamin D analogue,* directly lowers PTH levels. It can increase blood phosphorus and calcium levels, though, so calcium and phosphorus are monitored closely during use of this medication. If you are receiving treatment at a dialysis center, you will probably be provided with a vitamin D analogue such as Zemplar (paricalcitol) or Hectorol (doxercalciferol) intravenously as part of your treatment. If you are on home HD or peritoneal dialysis, you will probably take an oral form of the medication once or several times a week, depending on your level of PTH. Zemplar and Hectorol are also available as capsules, and Rocaltrol (calcitriol) can be taken in the form of capsules or an oral solution.

The most common side effects of activated vitamin D use are dizziness, lightheadedness, and nausea. Side effects that are possible but very rare include allergic symptoms such as rash, hives, swelling of the lips or tongue, or difficulty breathing; and chest pain or palpitations. Notify your doctor if you experience any of these symptoms.

A relatively new innovation in the treatment of hyperparathyroidism is the drug Sensipar (cinacalcet). This drug is a *calcimimetic*, which means that it mimics the action of calcium on the parathyroid gland, thereby signaling the gland to produce less PTH. As a result, serum calcium and phosphorus levels may also become more normal. If you have low calcium, though, you may not be a candidate for this medication as it may further lower your calcium levels.

Available in tablet form, Sensipar should be taken once a day with dinner. Swallow the pill whole; do not crush or break it. If you forget to take a dose, skip it and take the usual dose (not a double dose) the next day. Sensipar may cause nausea and stomach upset. Call your doctor immediately if you have a serious side effect such as numbness or tightness around your mouth, changed heart rate, muscle tightness or contraction, shortness of breath, or seizures.

THAT'S A LOT OF MEDICATION!

The number of pills that you will have to take each day will depend not only on your blood work, but also on whether you're getting treatments at home or at a dedicated center. If you're being dialyzed at a center, some of your meds will be provided intravenously.

It certainly can be a challenge to take all of those medications, especially when it comes to the phosphorus binders, which are often needed in quantity. The following tips can help you stay on top of your medication schedule and avoid missed or extra doses:

• Use a divided medication box—available at most drugstores—to put each day's pills in one place. This will not only help you remember your meds but will also mean that most of your pill bottles will have to be opened only one day a week, when you fill the box. Whenever you can't remember whether you took a pill, you'll be able to find out quickly by looking at that day's compartment.

- Make your medications a regular part of your everyday routine. For instance, decide that you're going to take your morning meds right after you brush your teeth. After a couple of weeks, this will be a habit.

- As necessary, use visual and auditory reminders to keep on track. Post-It notes stuck to the refrigerator and digital watches or cell phones programmed to beep at set times are all good ways to remind yourself to take your meds.

- If you find that you never have your phosphorus binders with you when you need them, fill several small containers (clearly marked) with the binders and keep one in the kitchen, one in your coat pocket or purse, one at work, and one in the car. That way, you'll always have these important pills on hand.

Make yourself as familiar as possible with your medications, and always keep a current list of your meds, including the purpose of each one. Take the list with you when you visit your nephrologist or other doctor so that if he makes a change in your drug schedule, you'll be able to mark it directly on the list.

IN CONCLUSION

Dialysis patients who are active participants in their medical care—who are aware of their blood work trends, who understand their medications, and who take their medications as prescribed—are likely to feel better. If you're not sure why a drug is being prescribed or why the dosage has been adjusted, by all means, ask your nephrologist or nurse for an explanation. The more you know, the more successfully you'll be able to follow and benefit from your regimen.

PART TWO

$\mathcal{T}$aking Action

In Part One, you learned the basics of dialysis—what it is, how it works, and which lab tests and medications are associated with the treatment process. Now it's time to go beyond the fundamentals and take action. Part Two explores different aspects of treatment and presents a wealth of positive steps you can take to maximize your health. I believe that the actions you take and the decisions you make can be the difference between surviving and thriving on dialysis.

Chapter 6 examines two crucial dialysis issues—fluid balance and blood pressure. Understanding these aspects of treatment and doing everything you can to take control of them can have an enormous effect on the way you feel and how you respond to dialysis. You'll learn why fluid balance and blood pressure are so important, and you'll discover how to pay attention to the way your body feels as a means of monitoring the effects your treatments are having on your body.

In Chapter 5, you learned about the medications you may be given *because* you are on dialysis. But there are a number of meds you may be taking for other disorders, as well. Chapter 7 focuses on the prescription drugs that are required for the treatment of three common health problems—diabetes, infection, and high blood pressure. Most important, it looks at how your body's reaction to them can be affected by kidney failure and dialysis. Dialysis does complicate the use of pharmaceuticals, but by understanding this aspect of care, asking the right questions of your doctor, and listening to your body, you can help insure that all of your medications are used both safely and effectively.

When you are on dialysis, a number of factors—including the dialysis process itself—can contribute to nutritional deficiencies. The renal vitamins discussed in Chapter 5 address only some of these health problems. In Chapter 8, you will learn about additional supplements that can enhance your energy, combat inflammation, support bone health, protect your cardiovascular system, and even assist your body in eliminating those toxins that are not removed by dialysis.

You probably already know that chronic kidney disease places limits on your diet, but are you aware that dialysis creates special dietary needs? Chapter 9 looks at the different components of a healthy dialysis diet, highlighting those nutrients that should be limited as well as those that you may have to consume in greater quantity because of your treatments. Food lists guide you to the best choices, and suggested menus help take the guesswork out of meal planning. Just as important, throughout the chapter, you will learn how diet can be used to improve overall health.

If you want to feel your best, you have to take care of not just your physical body, but also your mental and spiritual well-being. Chapter 10 addresses all three aspects of your health and offers proven ways in which you can strengthen your muscles and cardiovascular system, boost your energy, cultivate and maintain a positive frame of mind, and keep yourself strong and motivated even when life gets tough. Can meditation, prayer, and exercise actually help you do better on dialysis? They can, and this chapter will show you how it's done.

For many people, dialysis is a bridge to transplantation, which is considered the gold standard of treatment. If you are one of the thousands of people for whom transplantation is a possibility, Chapter 11 will be of interest to you. It starts by outlining some fundamentals of transplantation and then explains the process through which every potential candidate is evaluated. It also makes you aware of a relatively new program that is helping thousands of people get a new lease on life.

By the time you reach Chapter 12, you will have learned dozens of ways in which you can improve your health. While all of these tips and guidelines are important, I know they can be a bit overwhelming. That's why this chapter focuses on ten important ways in which you can help yourself feel better both during and between dialysis treatments. A special discussion suggests activities that can enable you to avoid boredom during those long treatment sessions.

Are you ready to take action? The following chapters will hand you the reins of your treatment so that you can improve your dialysis, enhance your overall health, and make every day of your life fuller and more enjoyable.

6

Controlling Fluid Balance and Blood Pressure

As you learned in Chapter 1, one of the most vital jobs performed by healthy kidneys is the regulation of body fluids. Functioning kidneys constantly monitor the fluid in the body and adjust the amounts of urine and sweat that are excreted so that the body retains the precise amount of fluid it needs to function, no more and no less. When the kidneys fail, dialysis has to take on the job of eliminating excess fluids. The problem is that while healthy kidneys work twenty-four hours a day, seven days a week, dialysis treatments are performed only a few hours a week. This means that fluids can build up between treatments, resulting in a number of health conditions, including high blood pressure. Then, during the dialysis treatment, any excess fluid is removed from the body. But if too much is removed, other problems can result, including *low* blood pressure.

As you can see, dialysis is a balancing act. Ideally, it should remove the excess fluid from your body without removing so much that you actually become dehydrated. If you have hemodialysis in a dedicated facility, your dialysis team will do its best to set the machine so that it will filter out the right amount of fluids, but it's important to understand that you, as the patient, need to play a role in controlling your fluid balance and blood pressure. That's why this chapter was written. First, it will explain the issue of fluid balance so that you understand it. This issue is often intertwined with blood pressure (BP) problems, but in some cases, these problems can occur for other reasons, so we'll cover that too. Finally, you will find tips and strategies for controlling fluid buildup between treatments and avoiding fluid- and blood pressure-related problems during the process of dialysis.

One important point should be made before you start learning about fluid balance and blood pressure. Although these issues are of some concern to all dialysis patients, they are of greatest concern to people who have three-times-a-week in-center hemodialysis (HD). People who use peritoneal dialysis (PD), are on home HD, or who have frequent nocturnal HD tend to have better-controlled fluid levels and blood pressure due to either increased treatment duration (nocturnal HD) or increased treatment frequency (home HD and PD).

KEEPING THE RIGHT FLUID BALANCE

Even if you've only read the introduction to this chapter, you understand that the control of body fluid levels is a bit complicated—but vitally important. You see, excess fluid gains can cause real problems. Let's begin our discussion by looking at the health risks of excess body fluid.

What Are the Effects of Excess Fluid?

In Chapter 1, we discussed the problems caused by the body's retention of fluid, but because we're now addressing the issue of fluid balance, it's important to briefly look at this topic again. Excess fluid retention can potentially cause:

- Temporary weight gain
- High blood pressure due to excess fluid in the bloodstream
- *Edema*, or swelling, usually seen in the feet, ankles, wrists, and face
- Bloating of the abdomen
- Shortness of breath due to fluid in the lungs
- Heart problems such as congestive heart failure (CHF)

It's worth mentioning that although excess fluids always cause temporary weight gain, the other problems listed above don't occur in all dialysis patients. By keeping excess fluid gain to a minimum and going for scheduled dialysis treatments, you can help avoid complications due to chronic excess fluids.

How Much Fluid
Needs to Be Removed by Dialysis?

As explained in Chapter 2, the excess fluid that builds up between treatments—as well as excess sodium—is removed during dialysis by a process called *ultrafiltration* (see the inset on page 20). In hemodialysis, the machine is set so that it continues to remove fluids until the person reaches her *estimated dry weight* (or *EDW*). This term is used to describe your weight without excess fluids. It's similar to what a person with healthy kidney function would weigh after getting rid of excess fluids (called *fluid weight*) through urination. To put it another way, your estimaed dry weight is the weight at which no more fluids can be removed without creating low blood pressure.

There is no way of scientifically measuring dry weight, so it is estimated by your doctor based on your weight during the following circumstances:

- You have normal blood pressure.
- You have no signs of edema.
- You have no shortness of breath.
- You have an absence of lung sounds that can be related to excess fluid.

Generally, an individual's dry weight is determined by trial and error. Every time you go for a dialysis treatment, you are weighed. This weight, as well as the EDW, is expressed in kilograms. (See the inset on page 80 to learn about kilograms.) The difference between your pre-treatment weight and your EDW is considered fluid weight, and the dialysis machine is set to remove that excess fluid and restore the estimated dry weight. As mentioned earlier, this is a balancing act. The healthcare team tries to minimize the problems associated with excess fluid between treatments, and minimize the problems associated with the removal of too much fluid during treatments.

What can happen if dialysis removes too much water and you go below your true dry weight? This can result in dehydration and the following problems:

- Thirst
- Uncomfortably dry mouth
- Muscle cramping
- Lightheadedness
- Nausea
- Rapid heartbeat
- Coldness in extremities

The amount of excess fluid is dynamic and can change from day to day and week to week, depending on how much you drink and how much sodium you consume. (You'll learn more about sodium on page 82.) Your estimated dry weight can also change—although it does so more gradually—due to dieting, decreased eating, or increased eating. Moreover, if you are wearing more or less clothing than usual at your weigh-in, your water weight may appear to be higher or lower than it really is. That's why, during the dialysis process, your dialysis team will ask you how you're feeling as one means of determining if the estimated dry weight and the estimated water weight are accurate. If you feel bad—if you are experiencing cramping or you feel dizzy or lightheaded—this is a subjective sign that too much fluid is being removed and that the setting should be changed on the dialysis machine. If your blood pressure gets really low during treatments, this may be an objective sign that too much

What Are Kilograms?

When you're on dialysis, your team will measure your weight in kilograms (kg) instead of pounds. Kilograms, as you know, are metric units, and if it makes you feel any better, physicians hate them, too. It may take you a while to get used to thinking in terms of kilograms, but the conversion of kilograms to pounds is really pretty simple: 1 kilogram equals 2.2 pounds, 2 kilograms equal 4.4 pounds, etc.

How much fluid are you likely to gain between treatments? This varies widely among patients, but for an average-sized person, the goal is generally to keep fluid weight gain at or below 1 kilogram, or 2.2 pounds, per day. This means that when there are two days between treatments, the goal is to gain less than 2 kilograms, or 4.4 pounds, in fluid. Of course, your individual goal for weight gain between treatments must be determined by your nephrologist.

fluid is being removed. (As you'll learn later in the chapter, low blood pressure is not always a sign of dehydration.) The way you feel at the *end* of dialysis is also important. If you experience dizziness and exhaustion, again, it may mean that too much fluid is being removed. Sometimes, changing your dry weight so that .5 kilogram (about 1 pound) less is filtered out can make a huge difference in the way you feel. Let your dialysis team know about your body's response to the treatment so they can consider if modifying your dry weight would be of benefit to you.

At the beginning of the chapter, I mentioned that fluid balance is most difficult for patients on standard in-center hemodialysis, and this fact deserves to be discussed in a little more detail. As you know, standard in-center hemodialysis (first explained on page 22), is usually done three times a week for about four hours. This means that fluids build up on the days between treatments and have to be removed during a four-hour period. Nocturnal hemodialysis (first discussed on page 23) is performed three nights a week for six to eight hours at a time, so you not only get a more thorough elimination of toxins, but also more time for excess fluids to be removed. Home HD (page 24) usually involves four or five dialysis sessions per week, so it also does a better job than standard HD of minimizing fluid gains between treatments. With peritoneal dialysis (page 25), there are either long periods of dialysis throughout the day or, if you're using a cycler, a gradual elimination of fluids overnight. And by using different dialysis solutions, you can more or less control the amount of fluids you lose. To put it simply, more frequent dialysis and longer dialysis means less fluid buildup, fewer fluid-related problems, and fewer dialysis-related blood pressure extremes.

Because significant gains and losses of fluid weight can be traumatic to the body, all dialysis patients—but especially three-times-a-week HD patients—should gain as little fluid as possible between treatments. That's why the next section focuses on minimizing fluid gain.

How Can You Reduce Fluid Gain?

Because people on dialysis know that fluid control is essential, one of the most frequent questions I'm asked by my patients is, "How much water can I drink?" It's important to realize that the total amount of fluid you gain does not result solely from the water you drink, but also from the salt you consume. Moreover, you'll want to make sure to consume high-quality liquids.

First, let's talk about salt, or sodium. (See the inset below to learn the difference between the two substances.) Sodium causes the body to retain more fluid and also increases your thirst so that you want to drink more. In general, you should restrict your sodium intake to no more than 2,000 mg (milligrams) a day. If you can, try to consume no more than 1,500 mg of sodium a day. If you are on home HD, nocturnal HD, or PD, you can be on the higher end of this sodium restriction—in other words, about 2,000 mg per day—because your treatments help prevent an excessive buildup of fluids. If you are on three-times-a-week in-center dialysis, you really have to be more strict—no more than 1,500 mg a day. Realize, though, that these are general guidelines. Don't hesitate to speak to your renal dietitian about your specific sodium restrictions.

Now let's talk about fluid restrictions. In general, it is recommended that dialysis patients drink no more than four to five cups a day (a quart to a quart plus one cup). But this limit can, in fact, be affected by several factors. Even though you are on dialysis, you may still have some residual kidney function, which means that you may still be able to urinate. If

Is There a Difference Between Sodium and Salt?

People who are on dialysis—as well as people with high blood pressure—are always told to limit sodium or salt. Do these two terms describe the same substance, or is there a difference between sodium and salt?

Sodium is a mineral that's found naturally in many foods, from vegetables to meats. It is essential to life, but like many nutrients, it is not healthy when consumed in excess. The term *salt* actually refers to sodium chloride, a substance that is only 40 percent sodium and 60 percent chloride. If your healthcare provider tells you to limit you daily consumption to, say, 2,000 mg of sodium, she's talking about pure sodium. Of course, you have to control your use of salt, too, because table salt is 40 percent sodium. If you do use salt in cooking or at the table, just remember that $\frac{1}{4}$ teaspoon of salt is the equivalent of 600 mg of sodium, and therefore will use up a good part of your daily sodium budget.

so, you will be able to drink more than people who have no kidney function. This also means that you may be able to take diuretics, which can help your body rid itself of more fluids. (You'll learn more about diuretics on page 97 of Chapter 7.) And, of course, if you are on nocturnal HD, home HD, or PD, you will be able to drink more because the dialysis will eliminate more fluids. The bottom line is that your healthcare team, and especially your dietitian, will determine your daily fluid allowance, and it is very important to follow the guidelines that are provided.

What Kind of Fluids Should You Drink?

Now that you know a little bit more about fluid limitations, you may be wondering what kind of fluids you should drink—as well as what kind you should avoid—on dialysis. First and foremost, I recommend eliminating any beverages that contain high-fructose corn syrup, phosphoric acid (which is a form of phosphorus), or artificial sweeteners, as well as beverages that are high in caffeine. This means skipping both regular and diet sodas—especially colas, which tend to be higher in phosphoric acid. Also avoid juices that are high in sugar or potassium. The latter includes orange, prune, and tomato juice.

Your best bet is to make high-quality water your drink of choice. Having good, safe drinking water is vital to everyone's health, but is especially important to those on dialysis because their body can't filter our impurities. You might be surprised by the number of impurities found in most tap water—metals such as cadmium, lead, and arsenic; bacteria; and even medications. While the long-term effects on humans are not known, they can't be good.

If you drink tap water, a good first step is to check your local drinking water by contacting your local water authority, which is required to provide an annual Consumer Confidence Report that lists the levels of all regulated contaminants. Bottled water is another good option as long as the plastic bottles are free of bisphenol A (BPA), which can leach into the water. Your best bet, though, is to purchase a filtration system which produces water that is not only free of contaminants, but also mildly alkaline. Alkaline water can help reduce the inflammatory response and control the hyperacidity that is often associated with kidney disease. (For more information on water filtration systems, see page 179 of the Resources section.)

Other than water, what beverages are both safe and beneficial? After a dialysis treatment, a glass of freshly made vegetable and fruit juice is a great way to benefit from the anti-inflammatory, antioxidant, alkaline effects of produce—as long as you avoid high-potassium foods. (See page 127 of Chapter 9 for lists of high- and low-potassium foods.) One good pick-me-up combination is kale, carrots, and apples. Put the produce in a juicer and you will be good to go. You can vary what you include in the juice drink depending on your potassium restrictions, but I would recommend only one fruit per drink—in most cases, an apple, lemon, or lime. Many other fruits are more acidic.

You can enjoy vegetable juices even if you have severe fluid restrictions. For example, a four- or eight-ounce glass of freshly made juice is perfectly fine in the morning. For some, it can even take the place of breakfast foods. Freshly made vegetable juices are a great way to supplement much-needed nutrients when you don't feel like eating.

Another good choice is green tea. It is high in health-promoting antioxidants, especially epigallocatechin gallate (EGCG), and low in caf-

Understanding Blood Pressure Readings

Most people have blood pressure problems when they begin dialysis, and their BP remains a significant issue throughout their years of treatment. What is blood pressure and what do the readings mean? That's what this inset was designed to explain.

Blood pressure is the pressure your blood exerts against your blood vessels as your heart pumps blood. Each reading is made up of two numbers. The top number, which is also the higher of the two numbers, is called the *systolic pressure.* It measures the pressure in the arteries at the peak of a heartbeat, when the heart muscle contracts. The bottom number, which is also the lower of the two numbers, refers to the *diastolic pressure.* It measures the pressure in the arteries between the heartbeats, when the heart muscle is relaxing and refilling with blood. Therefore, the reading 140/90 mmHg (millimeters of mercury) indicates a systolic pressure of 140 and a diastolic pressure of 90. Many feel that 140/90 is the goal blood pressure for a person on dialysis, but the "best" BP can be different for different dialysis patients. (To read more about this, see page 94 of Chapter 7.)

feine compared with coffee. Try to include eight ounces of this wonderful beverage in your daily fluid program.

UNDERSTANDING DIALYSIS-RELATED BLOOD PRESSURE CHANGES

Keeping blood pressure (BP) in an acceptable range can be a real battle for people on dialysis. As you now know, a lot of BP issues are directly tied to fluid volume. If you have excess fluid on board, this can raise your blood pressure. If you have a lot of fluid removed during dialysis, this can lower your blood pressure. But excess fluid and dehydration aren't the only reasons why blood pressure can get too high or low. Other possible causes include actions of the autonomic nervous system and heart problems. Below, you'll learn a little about each of these so that you can better understand blood pressure issues that may arise during dialysis.

The Autonomic Nervous System

Your *autonomic nervous* system, which is comprised of your *sympathetic* and *parasympathetic nervous systems,* helps control functions throughout your body, so it's no surprise that it's a major player in the control of blood pressure. When your blood pressure falls too low—or when your body needs higher blood pressure to deal with a physical threat—the sympathetic part of the system uses chemical messengers to speed up your heartbeat and raise your blood pressure. (Think of what happens during the "fight or flight" reaction to physical threats.) When your blood pressure gets too high—or when it's time for you to sleep—the parasympathetic system releases chemicals that slow down your heart and lower your blood pressure.

We don't know why, but in some people, dialysis seems to trigger autonomic nervous system-related changes in blood pressure. Some people have good blood pressure until they start a dialysis treatment. Then their blood pressure goes through the roof for no apparent reason, and changing the setting on the dialysis machine to remove more fluids doesn't seem to help. Other people may start a dialysis treatment only to have their BP drop—again, for no apparent reason. Sometimes the blood pressure rises again after treatment ends, and sometimes it remains low.

If your blood pressure rises or drops during dialysis, and this response does not seem directly related to fluids, speak to your doctor to explore other possibilities. If it seems that the problem may be associated with the autonomic nervous system, a change may have to be made in any blood pressure medications you're taking.

If your blood pressure tends to drop during dialysis, on treatment days, you may have to avoid taking BP meds. Your doctor may also prescribe a medication like ProAmatine (midodrine hydrochloride), which raises blood pressure.

If your blood pressure tends to rise at the beginning of a dialysis treatment, consider if it may be related to the pain you experience when needles are inserted in your access. Pain can definitely cause an increase in BP, so if it's a problem for you, ask your dialysis nurse or technician to use a topical anesthetic cream or spray on your skin before inserting the needles. It may do the trick. Blood pressure can also be affected by anxiety. If you feel apprehensive at the beginning of a treatment, try starting the session with a period of deep breathing, meditation, or visualization of a successful dialysis session. (To learn a simple deep breathing exercise, see page 139.) Several of my patients have found these practices very effective in controlling dialysis-related hypertension. If these strategies don't help, your doctor may have to prescribe an ACE inhibitor or beta blocker to keep your blood pressure from rising. (You'll learn more about blood pressure medications in Chapter 7.)

Heart and Valve Problems

As mentioned earlier, dialysis-related blood pressure problems can also be caused by heart problems. For instance, *aortic stenosis,* a condition in which the opening of the aortic valve is narrowed, can make it difficult for the heart to pump blood to the rest of the body. It's like trying to make water flow through a garden hose that has a kink in it. Then, if too much fluid is pulled out of the bloodstream during dialysis, aortic stenosis can cause a significant lowering of blood pressure. Aortic stenosis, as well as other heart valve problems, can be assessed with an *echocardiogram,* which uses sound waves to create a moving picture of your heart. Surgery is sometimes required to relieve this problem so that dialysis can be used without causing a drop in blood pressure.

As first discussed in Chapter 1, *congestive heart failure,* or *CHF,* is a condition in which the heart can no longer pump blood to the rest of the body either because it is too weak to pump well (*systolic failure*) or because it is too stiff to relax (*diastolic failure*). If you have been diagnosed with CHF, it is especially important to watch your fluid intake and fluid gain between treatments. Some people with advanced CHF run a lower-than-normal blood pressure all the time—even when not on dialysis. Fortunately, the proper medication can help. Your doctor may prescribe beta blockers or ACE inhibitors, which can help normalize blood pressure and also be heart-protective. (To learn more about medications used to treat blood pressure, see page 94 of Chapter 7.)

TIPS FOR CONTROLLING FLUID BALANCE AND BLOOD PRESSURE

Being a dialysis patient is a full-time job. You have to be an active participant in your own healthcare and do what you can to avoid between-treatment fluid gains and related blood pressure extremes, as well as fluid- and blood-pressure-associated problems that can occur during dialysis therapy. The following tips can help you take charge.

• Bug your dietitian for all the information you need to control fluid gain. Ask her what your fluid and sodium limits are, and request lists of beverages and other foods that should be avoided because of high sodium levels. If you want additional information, check the Internet, where you'll find a lot of great data on foods. For instance, the National Kidney Foundation's website provides a wealth of nutritional information specifically designed for kidney patients, and the site Self Nutrition Data can generate lists of foods that are high and low in particular nutrients. (See pages 178 and 179 of the Resources section for contact information.)

• Be an informed consumer and check the sodium information listed on food labels when you do your grocery shopping. Pay attention to portion size so that you know how much sodium is in the amount of food that you actually eat or drink. While one portion may be okay, a whole package may provide more of this mineral than you should have. (See page 124 for a guide to reading food labels.)

- To make sure that you stick to your daily fluid limits, pre-fill a pitcher with the total amount of fluid that you are allowed to drink, or, if you spend a lot of time away from home, take along the exact amount of bottled water that you are allowed to have.

- Do what you can to make sure that your pre-dialysis weigh-in is as accurate as possible and won't lead the dialysis team to miscalculate your fluid weight. Take off your coat before getting up on the scale. It's fine to wear shoes for the weigh-in, but try to wear the same type of shoes every week, because clunky shoes and big boots can make a huge difference. Did you put on an extra sweater this morning? If you don't usually wear that much clothing for your weigh-ins, shed the extra garment before you weigh yourself.

- Tell your dialysis team if you think that your dry weight—your "real" weight, without excess fluids—might have changed significantly since your last treatment. If you've been eating less food than usual because of illness, for instance, let your team know.

- If significant changes in blood pressure take place during dialysis treatments, and these changes don't seem to be a response to the elimination of fluids, speak to your doctor about other potential causes. Possibly, a change in medication on the day of dialysis or the treatment of an underlying problem can better control your blood pressure, both during and between dialysis sessions.

IN CONCLUSION

To thrive on dialysis, you must do whatever you can to control fluid gains between treatments; remain aware of your "dialysis vital signs," which include blood pressure and dry weight; and be your own patient advocate. Don't be afraid to ask questions of your team or to even suggest different strategies, and don't hesitate to tell them how you're feeling during and between treatments—something that you know way better than any doctor does. Perhaps by simply tweaking your dry weight or changing a medication, your team will be able to turn uncomfortable dialysis sessions into much more pleasant experiences, and even improve your well-being between treatments.

7

*T*aking Other Medications on Dialysis

When most medications are taken, they are absorbed into the bloodstream; delivered to the target cells, tissues, or organs; and metabolized (processed) through the liver. Then, the components that are not used by the body are excreted, usually through the kidneys. It is these steps that determine how long the medication or its metabolites (the products of its metabolism) remain active in the body.

When the kidneys have very limited function or have completely ceased to function, as is true in the case of dialysis patients, the way that certain drugs work is affected. Many drugs, for instance, tend to stay in the body for a greater length of time. Moreover, the process of dialysis itself can filter out medications while they are still in the bloodstream, so that they don't have a chance to do their job. Dialysis can even affect the condition for which the medication has been prescribed.

This doesn't mean that you can't take blood pressure drugs, diabetic medications, and other pharmaceuticals that are required for your health, but it does mean that the specific drugs used, the dosage, and/or the dosage schedule may have to be changed when you begin dialysis. This chapter focuses on the medications that are most commonly prescribed not because you are on dialysis—those drugs are covered in Chapter 5—but because you have another health disorder, such as diabetes, infection, or high blood pressure. The more you know and understand about the medications you are taking and the way they may be affected by kidney failure and dialysis, the better you will be able to actively participate in your own healthcare.

DIABETES MEDICATIONS

Diabetes is the most common cause of kidney failure, accounting for nearly 44 percent of new cases. For this reason, the control of blood glucose levels is an important issue for many dialysis patients.

Diabetes is a chronic condition in which the body's insufficient secretion of the hormone insulin or its inability to use insulin leads to excessive amounts of glucose (sugar) in the blood. Anti-diabetes medications are used to lower blood glucose to normal levels. Unfortunately, both kidney failure (specifically, uremia, discussed on page 10) and dialysis have an impact on blood glucose levels. In fact, they have opposite effects, causing blood glucose levels to fluctuate widely. In addition, because most diabetes drugs are at least partially excreted by the kidneys, the drugs tend to stay in the body for a longer period of time than they should and increase the risk of *hypoglycemia*, or low blood sugar. As you can imagine, all of these factors complicate the control of glucose levels, which is at the heart of diabetes management.

Insulin, which is taken intravenously, is considered a cornerstone of diabetes treatment. But even insulin can stay in the body longer than it would in people with functioning kidneys and put you at greater risk for hypoglycemia. Understand, too, that the time you spend in dialysis treatments can delay meals, causing blood sugar levels to drop. (See the inset on page 92 to learn more about this.) This is why doses of insulin usually must be lowered for dialysis patients, and doses must be timed carefully, as well.

Some oral diabetes drugs can be used by people who are on dialysis, but some must be strictly avoided. For instance, Amaryl (glimeripiride), which belongs to the sulfonylureas class of oral diabetes medications, depends on the kidneys for excretion, so it can remain in the body longer. Although it can be used by dialysis patients, the dosage must be modified to take its longer action into consideration. Glucophage (metformin), on the other hand, should *never* be used by people with advanced kidney disease, whether or not they are on dialysis. The take-home message is clear: Both kidney disease and dialysis affect the way the body reacts to diabetes medications. It's vital to be aware of your glucose levels, to let your endocrinologist know that you are on dialysis, and to okay your diabetes medications with your nephrologist. If your blood sugar levels are not being well controlled, the dose of your medication may have to be changed or the medication you're taking may have to be replaced with an entirely different drug.

Of course, you will feel better if you do all that you can to keep your glucose levels within a healthy range. The following tips should help:

- Do your best to eat three meals a day, plus a few snacks, and avoid foods high in sugar. This will help prevent your blood sugar from fluctuating too much. Your dietitian will tell you which foods are best for you and which should be avoided.

- Talk to your dietitian about planning meals around dialysis times. If you have dialysis on some days only—if you are on hemodialysis, in other words—be sure to create meal plans for both dialysis days and non-dialysis days. If you can, try to eat in the morning before your dialysis, especially if you have an early morning shift at a dialysis center. This can decrease the risk of experiencing hypoglycemia during your session. Then take along a healthful snack that can be eaten at the end of your treatment.

- Check your blood sugar as often as your doctor prescribes, and check it more frequently on dialysis days. Remember that the combination of kidney disease and dialysis can make blood sugar levels jump up and down.

- Discuss the timing of your medications with your doctor, and explore the possibility of changing the dose on dialysis days. Then take the medications exactly as prescribed.

ANTIBIOTICS

Antibiotics—medications used to treat bacterial infections—are another type of drug that may be given to dialysis patients. Sometimes, they are prescribed for dialysis-related problems such as catheter infections. Sometimes, they are prescribed for disorders that are not directly related to kidney failure or dialysis, such as sore throat, upper respiratory tract infection, and/or bronchitis.

Antibiotics have to be chosen carefully for the dialysis patient. Some commonly prescribed antibiotics, such as Macrodantin (nitrofurantoin)

How "True" Hemodialysis Time Affects Blood Sugar Levels

If you have already begun standard hemodialysis treatments in a dedicated center, and you also have diabetes, you know what your dialysis days are like. Perhaps you take your diabetes medication in the morning. Then you have to drive or take a transport service to your dialysis center. The trip itself probably takes you from thirty minutes to an hour. When you arrive, you first get weighed in; then you wait a little longer before the session starts. The treatment lasts from three to four hours, but there's probably further delay before you're completely unhooked from the machine. Finally, you travel home—another thirty minutes to an hour.

The long stretch between the time you leave home and the time you return home—a stretch during which you go without food—can result in low blood glucose (hypoglycemia) and associated symptoms such as nausea, nervousness, rapid heartbeat, and trembling. If you feel sick at the end of your session, you may not even want to eat when you get home. There may be other complications, as well, such as diabetic *gastroparesis (gas-tro-par-ee-sis),* a slowing of the digestive system. In other words, on treatment days, you may be going without food longer than you realize.

How can you keep your blood sugar as even as possible on days like this? The first step is to be aware of how your body reacts to both dialysis and medications. This means taking your blood glucose levels both before and after a dialysis session. If the levels are not being well controlled, talk with your nephrologist or endocrinologist about changing the dose of your medication or even skipping a dose on the morning before dialysis. A different timing and dose can made a big difference in the way you feel. Also speak to your dietitian about scheduling meals and snacks for better diabetes management. (See page 91 for more tips on controlling blood sugar.)

and Bactrim (sulfamethoxazole and trimethoprim), should be avoided on dialysis if at all possible. Other drugs, like Levaquin (levofloxacin), can be used, but the usual dosage schedule should be modified. Like the medications used to control diabetes, antibiotics are normally metabolized in the liver and eliminated through the kidneys. When kidney function is severely reduced, these drugs stay active in the body longer. If the antibiotic is not dosed properly, potentially bad side effects can occur. Certain types of antibiotics can cause confusion or even seizures if the dosage is not appropriate. On the other hand, the process of dialysis can actually remove many antibiotics from the system before they work. In this case, the medication must be taken after the dialysis session is over.

Be aware that antibiotics are sometimes given intravenously as part of a hemodialysis treatment. This is commonly done in the case of catheter-related infections. Because dialysis can filter these medications out of your blood before they can take effect, they are generally given as late as possible during treatment, or even after treatment, depending on the drug being used. Every dialysis center has its own protocol regarding the timing of the dose.

A final point should be made about the use of antibiotics—and this is true for everyone and not just people on dialysis. While often needed to kill harmful "bugs," antibiotics can also kill the "friendly" bacteria in your bowels and cause problems such as diarrhea. That is why I recommend that when anyone takes a course of antibiotics, he should also take a probiotic. (See the inset on page 95 for more information.)

Considering the potential side effects of antibiotic use and the special needs of dialysis patients, it makes sense to avoid taking antibiotics when they are not necessary and to take precautions when they are prescribed. The following recommendations should help:

- To avoid access-related infections, follow the access-care guidelines provided on pages 44 to 47 of Chapter 3. As you learned in Chapter 3, hemodialysis and peritoneal dialysis catheters are more prone to infection than fistulas and grafts, so if you have a catheter, you should be especially vigilant in your care.

- Don't pressure your doctor to prescribe an antibiotic. Remember that antibiotics treat bacterial infections, not viral infections, so they won't be effective against the common cold, the flu, most coughs, and minor sore throats. If you take antibiotics when you don't need them, you can develop drug-resistant bacteria that are difficult to treat.

- *Never* self-medicate by taking antibiotics that have been prescribed for someone else. They may be the wrong antibiotic and/or the wrong strength for you. This rule should be followed even by people who do not have chronic health problems, but it is especially important for people who are on dialysis.

• Whenever you receive a prescription for antibiotics, make sure that the drug can be taken by someone on dialysis and that the dosage has been adjusted with your condition in mind. If a physician other than your nephrologist prescribes an antibiotic—or any medication, for that matter—be sure to check it out with your kidney doctor to see if it's okay. Then follow the dosing directions carefully.

BLOOD PRESSURE MEDICATIONS

As much as 80 percent of people with chronic kidney disease have high blood pressure, or *hypertension.* In fact, most people are already taking blood pressure-lowering medication, called *antihypertensives,* when they begin dialysis treatments. But as you learned in Chapter 6, it can be a challenge for the dialysis patient to keep blood pressure within a healthy range. Between treatments, fluids can build up in the body, causing your blood pressure to rise. When these fluids are dialyzed out of the body, blood pressure can actually become too low—especially during hemodialysis, which rapidly removes a great quantity of fluids. So your doctor will have to take special care to prescribe the right blood pressure med for you and to administer it at the right times so that it will not lead to *hypotension* (low blood pressure) and will not be filtered out of your blood before it has its intended effect.

Is there an ideal blood pressure for someone who undergoes dialysis? In Chapter 6, I mentioned that many nephrologists aim for a goal blood pressure of 140/90 mmHg or less. (See the inset on page 84 for an explanation of blood pressure readings.) That being said, as of yet, there is no "official" goal BP. Just as important, some people feel better with slightly higher blood pressure—150/90 mmHg, for instance—while others feel better at a lower blood pressure. Also, a higher-than-normal blood pressure may be desirable in a patient who has narrowing of the carotid artery, or *carotid stenosis.* In other words, while there are general blood pressure guidelines for people on dialysis, your doctor has to personalize your medication regimen based on your health condition and how you feel.

Understanding Antibiotics and Intestinal Health

When bacterial infections occur, antibiotics are usually the treatment of choice. Unfortunately, while these medications can do a great job of killing off the "bad bacteria" that caused the infection, they can also destroy the so-called "good bacteria." Most important, they can do real damage to the colonies of beneficial flora that populate the bowel. Since these bacteria perform a host of important functions—from digesting food to producing vitamin K to supporting the body's immune system— a course of antibiotics can result in some nasty side effects, including diarrhea, bloody stool, bloating, and vaginal yeast infections. In the worst case scenario, the repeated use of antibiotics or a single course of certain antibiotics can lead to the potentially devastating intestinal infection known as *Clostridium difficile colitis.*

I believe that everyone on dialysis, and even people with early-stage kidney disease, should be on *probiotics,* which are live cultures of bacteria that are normally found in the digestive system. When you are taking antibiotics, you should most certainly take a probiotic to prevent unpleasant and potentially dangerous side effects. To learn more about probiotic supplements, see page 108 of Chapter 8.

Just like antibiotics and diabetes medications, blood pressure meds have to be chosen and dosed carefully when someone is on dialysis, with full knowledge of how the drug can be affected by the dialysis treatment being used. For instance, Lopressor (metoprolol), a type of beta blocker, is removed by hemodialysis. The ACE inhibitor Altace (ramipril) is significantly removed by hemodialysis, while another drug in this class, Zestril (lisinopril), is only partially dialyzed out. On the other hand, many classes of antihypertensive medications—including angiotensin receptor blockers (ARBs) such as Diovan (valsartan) and Cozaar (losartan)—are *not* affected by hemodialysis. Some drugs, including calcium channel blocks such as Norvasc (amlodipine) and Calan (verapamil), may be more affected by peritoneal dialysis than they are by HD. The bottom line is that depending on the drug taken, the timing may have to be adjusted, especially on dialysis days. Usually, this means taking your medication after your dialysis session. In some cases, it may be best to switch to another medication entirely.

At this point, it's important to understand that every medication has a *half-life*—the time it takes for that particular drug to be eliminated from the bloodstream to half its strength. The ACE inhibitor Zestril (lisinopril), for instance, has a very long half-life; it takes about twelve hours for this drug to reach half-strength in the body. This is another factor that should be considered when medications are prescribed. When using a drug with a longer half-life, a three-times-a-week regimen may be best. In fact, this dosage schedule seems to work for a great many patients on blood pressure medication. (See the inset below.)

Another important factor that is considered when choosing an antihypertensive is the presence of health disorders other than kidney disease and hypertension. For instance, if at all possible, most kidney specialists prescribe ACE inhibitors and/or ARBs for their patients on dialysis, because these classes of medication are good for the heart in addition to helping control blood pressure. If a patient has congestive

Do Blood Pressure Medications Need to Be Given Every Day?

Doctors are trained to prescribe antihypertensive medications every day, the goal being to provide twenty-four-hour blood pressure control. But as you've learned, this type of schedule can sometimes cause excessively low blood pressure in dialysis patients. Because of this problem, one study examined a very small population of dialysis patients that were given antihypertensives three times a week. The specific medications included the long-acting blood pressure-lowering medications trandolapril, amlodipine, and atenolol. The patients in this study were initially started on trandolapril. If further blood pressure control was required, the other medications were added as needed.

At the end of the study, the three-times-a-week dosage was found to not only lower blood pressure, but also lower cost and pill burden to the patient. This novel approach provided a new way of treating hypertension while avoiding the blood pressure fluctuations often associated with dialysis treatments.

heart failure or a history of heart attack, a beta blocker may be pre-scribed, as well.

Because dialysis removes excess fluids from the body, your treat-ments may very well improve your high blood pressure, and eventually, may make antihypertensive drugs unnecessary. This is one reason why it's important to pay attention to the way your body is reacting to dial-ysis and to be aware of your blood pressure readings.

On page 87 of Chapter 6, I talk about some steps you can take to keep your blood pressure on track. It's worth repeating some of these guide-lines below and looking at some specific medication-related concerns:

- Between treatments, manage fluids as well as possible, following the guidelines provided on pages 78 to 85. This will help control your blood pressure both between and during dialysis sessions.

- Follow the diet prescribed by your dietitian and nephrologist. By carefully adhering to your diet, including the timing of meals, you will control fluid buildup and thus help avoid blood pressure highs and lows.

- During dialysis, be alert to symptoms of low blood pressure, includ-ing dizziness, nausea, headache, and muscle cramps. Immediately inform your team of these telltale signs.

- Talk to your doctor about your antihypertensive medication sched-ule. You'll want to discuss when you should take your meds on dial-ysis days versus non-dialysis days, and whether you should hold some medications until after your treatment. If you often have prob-lems with low blood pressure, ask your doctor if you can take your blood pressure meds every other day rather than every day.

- Once your medication schedule has been set, follow it exactly.

DIURETICS

Many dialysis patients still have significant *residual renal function (RRF)*, which means that they still have some ability to urinate even though their kidneys have lost the capacity to effectively filter out toxins. Despite this residual function, many of these people retain excess fluids between dialysis treatments. Fortunately, the use of *diuretics*—medications designed to increase the formation and discharge of urine—may help avoid excessive fluid buildup.

Certainly, anything that helps you minimize fluid gains is a plus, so if you still have some kidney function, you should speak to your doctor about the possibility of using diuretics. Some common options include Lasix (furosemide) and Demadex (torsemide). Just keep in mind that advanced kidney disease can cause the body to be diuretic-resistant, so you may need a higher-than-usual dose of the chosen medication.

As is true of many medications, the dosing schedule used for diuretics is very important. Although some physicians prescribe the daily use of these meds, this regimen can cause too much fluid loss on dialysis days. Some patients feel better when they take diuretics on non-dialysis days only.

Although diuretics can help you control unhealthy fluid gains, they should be used wisely to avoid problems. Here are a few tips:

- Even though you're using diuretics, be sure to follow the fluid and dietary guidelines provided by your nephrologist and dietitian. It's important to do everything possible to avoid fluid overload.

- Work with your doctor to determine the best schedule for taking diuretics. If you take diuretics on your dialysis days, you may end up removing too much fluid from your body. Usually, these drugs are used on non-dialysis days.

- Be alert for signs of low blood pressure, which can result from excess fluid loss. Symptoms—which can include dizziness, lightheadedness, nausea, headache, and muscle cramps—should be reported to your dialysis team.

- If you are experiencing vomiting or diarrhea, both of which cause fluid loss, check with your dialysis team before taking your diuretics. It may be a good idea to skip these medications until the vomiting or diarrhea stops.

- If you have residual kidney function, do whatever you can to protect it. The inset on page 99 will steer you away from some practices that can cause kidney function loss.

Preserving Residual Kidney Function

On page 97, you learned that many people who are on dialysis still have residual renal function (RRF). This is important because RRF has been shown to have many benefits, including, of course, better control of blood pressure and fluid volume through urination. You may have heard, though, that people tend to lose RRF when they're on dialysis, especially hemodialysis. This generally happens because the combination of blood pressure highs that occur between dialysis sessions and blood pressure lows that occur during sessions can cause a "stunning" of the kidneys. If the kidneys are stunned frequently over a period of time, you can lose whatever kidney function remains. In addition, certain drugs and procedures can damage kidney function.

Fortunately, there are steps you can take to maintain RRF:

- I've said it before, but it can't be overemphasized: *Avoid excessive fluid gain between treatments.* If your average between-treatment fluid gain is more than 3 kilograms (6.6 pounds), the removal of that fluid during a four-hour hemodialysis session will place a heck of a strain on your body and lead to a drop in blood pressure. By limiting fluid buildup through dietary and fluid restrictions, and possibly through the use of diuretics, you will help avoid dialysis-related kidney damage.

- Unless it is recommended by your nephrologist, try to avoid the dye used in some imaging studies, such as CT scans. These dyes can shut down the remaining few kidney cells that are functioning. This is not to say that you can never have this type of imaging, but you should permit it only when it's absolutely necessary. Be sure to talk to your doctor about possible safe non-dye alternatives.

- Exercise caution in the use of *nephrotoxic drugs*—drugs that can cause damage to the kidneys. Avoid more than occasional use of nonsteroidal anti-inflammatory drugs (NSAIDs), such as ibuprofen; the oral phosphate solutions used as purgatives before colonoscopies; and prolonged use of aminoglycoside antibiotics, such as streptomycin.

IN CONCLUSION

Always ask questions when you're prescribed a new medication to make sure that it is compatible with dialysis and that its dosing schedule will not in any way conflict with your treatment schedule. When a physician other than your nephrologist recommends a medication, discuss the prescription with your kidney doctor before filling it. Perhaps he will okay it, or perhaps he will contact your other physician to suggest switching to a different drug or changing the dose. I'm not kidding when I say that dialysis is a full-time job! You have to be your own advocate. The good news is that by becoming a well-informed participant in your own care, you will reap the benefits of better health and improved quality of life.

8

$\mathcal{U}$sing Nutritional Supplements on Dialysis

People who have chronic kidney disease (CKD) and are on dialysis are at risk of vitamin, mineral, and other nutrient deficiencies for several reasons. First, dialysis can rob your body of water-soluble nutrients such as the B vitamins. Second, advanced CKD causes abnormal renal metabolism and inadequate absorption of nutrients. Third, the dialysis diet limits the consumption of many foods, and people who have kidney failure and are on dialysis often have a poor appetite, as well, which prevents them from getting all the nutrients they need. Finally, the kidneys actually play a role in manufacturing some nutrients, so when these organs fail, you become deficient in those substances.

In Chapter 5, you learned that nephrologists usually prescribe renal vitamins for their patients. For the most part, these supplements provide the water-soluble vitamins that dialysis is prone to rob from the body, and they omit nutrients that can build up to dangerous levels in the bloodstream. That chapter also told you about activated vitamin D and iron—two nutrients that are given to most dialysis patients in the course of treatment. These pharmaceuticals are important, but in my practice, I have found that some additional supplements can be very helpful. When given judiciously, they can improve cell function, relieve some side effects of dialysis, alleviate nutritional deficiencies that are not addressed by renal vitamins, promote strong bones, reduce inflammation, and otherwise improve health and quality of life.

This chapter discusses a number of nutritional supplements that should be considered by everyone on dialysis. That being said, I have to add that this is a tricky topic because everyone's nutritional problems are different and everyone's health needs are unique. As you read about each of these potentially valuable supplements, keep in mind that no supplement should be taken without an okay from your nephrologist. Because she knows your blood work and is familiar with other health disorders you may have, she can best evaluate whether a nutrient would be beneficial or harmful to your health. She can also order additional tests to see whether you have certain nutritional deficiencies that could be relieved by supplementation.

SUPPLEMENTS THAT ENHANCE ENERGY AND PREVENT OXIDATIVE STRESS

One of the biggest complaints of people on dialysis is that that they are extremely fatigued. Both kidney disease and dialysis cause *oxidative stress.* This means that they promote the injury of cells by unstable molecules called *free radicals,* which are produced by the body as the result of normal physiological processes, chronic illness and inflammation, our toxic environment, and many other factors. This stress compromises cellular function, including the production of energy. In many cases, the resulting exhaustion is worsened by nutrient depletion, problems with blood pressure control, and other complications that are often associated with kidney disease and dialysis, as well as with common disorders like diabetes. Realize that dialysis, while it performs the important function of filtering the blood, can itself be a source of oxidative stress and inflammation.

The nutritional supplements discussed below supply antioxidants that can fight oxidative stress, enhance energy production, and, in some cases, also provide other important benefits.

Coenzyme Q_{10}

Coenzyme Q_{10}—also referred to as *CoQ_{10}* and *ubiquinone*—is a naturally occurring substance that is found throughout the body. (The word "ubiquinone" comes from "ubiquitous," which means, "found everywhere.") This substance plays an important role in producing energy in the mitochondria, which is the portion of the cell that generates a certain form of energy. If you have diabetes and are not on dialysis, your levels of CoQ_{10} are low. If you are on dialysis, your levels are, in fact, even lower. Infection and inflammation have also been found to reduce CoQ_{10}. Supplementation of this nutrient can help restore energy levels and also improve heart function.

I believe that everyone, whether or not they are on dialysis, should take CoQ_{10}. I generally recommend starting at 100 mg daily, and after several weeks, gradually increasing the dose to at least twice a day. For someone on dialysis, the upper limit is 200 to 300 mg a day. CoQ_{10} can be taken with or without food. On dialysis days, take this supplement after your treatment session. If you are on a statin medication or another med that can further deplete levels of this nutrient, the dose may have to be increased. CoQ_{10} can lower blood pressure in some people, so if your blood pressure tends to run low during dialysis treatments, you may have to start on a lower dose and increase slowly. This supplement can also lower blood sugar levels, so watch for this effect if blood sugar is a problem for you.

L-Carnitine

L-carnitine is an amino acid—a building block of protein—that is manufactured in the body. It is essential for the production of energy and important for heart function, muscle movement, and many other body processes. Because this substance is made in the liver and kidneys, kidney disease lowers the production of L-carnitine. Dialysis and a range of disorders also cause low levels of L-carnitine. Use of the supplement—which also has anti-inflammatory and antioxidant properties—can help restore healthy levels of the substance and improve energy. Supplementation can also help relieve the cramps that some people experience during dialysis. L-carnitine has heart-protective benefits, as well. Just as important, I believe that supplementation with L-carnitine is one of the keys to changing the body's chemistry from *catabolic* (a state of breaking down) to *anabolic* (a state of building up).

Please don't confuse the oral L-carnitine supplement with the intravenous form of the supplement. The IV form is used for a specific type of anemia that can accompany dialysis.

I recommend a starting dose of 500 mg of L-carnitine taken every other day. You can take this supplement either with meals or on an empty stomach. Slowly increase the dose with the goal of up to 1,000 mg a day.

D-Ribose

D-ribose occurs naturally in all living cells. A complex sugar, it begins the metabolic process that results in the production of adenosine triphosphate (ATP), an important energy-bearing molecule. D-ribose has been found to play a vital role in heart health and to be valuable in the treatment of heart problems such as congestive heart failure. When given to dialysis patients along with CoQ_{10} and L-carnitine, it improves energy levels, exercise capacity, and an overall sense of well-being. Although the nutrient is a sugar, it does not increase blood glucose levels. In fact, it can lower them.

D-ribose is available in both capsule and powder form. The powder is easier for some people to take because it can be mixed into green tea or another beverage. Both forms work well, though. If you wish to use the capsule form, take 2,000 to 2,500 mg every other day. If you prefer the powder, which is better tolerated than the capsules, take 2,500 every other day.

Alpha-Lipoic Acid

Also called *lipoic acid* and *thioctic acid, alpha-lipoic acid (ALA)* is a fatty acid that's naturally produced by the body. It is needed to convert glucose (blood sugar) into energy, and therefore helps maintain low blood sugar levels. It also appears to "recycle" antioxidants such as vitamin C and vitamin E after they have been used by the body. It can also increase the level of glutathione, which is one of the most potent antioxdiants of which we know. (You'll learn more about glutathione on page 106.)

Perhaps most important for the person on dialysis, this supplement has been found very helpful in treating *neuropathy*—a nerve disorder that can have many causes and appear in many forms. Dialysis itself can cause a type of neuropathy, and diabetes, too, can result in this disorder.

Can the Right Supplements Actually Relieve Fatigue?

A few years ago, one of my hemodialysis patients complained of extreme fatigue. She was so weak, tired, and drained that she didn't want to get out of bed. As you can imagine, her quality of life was extremely poor.

I quickly set to work. First, my team evaluated what she was eating and recommended that certain foods be added to her diet. Because she was reluctant to add too many pills to her regimen, I started her off on just three energy-boosting supplements—coenzyme Q_{10}, L-carnitine, and D-ribose. I began with low doses and increased slowly. Once she had adjusted to the supplements, I added alpha-lipoic acid. After a few weeks, my patient was a totally different person. Her energy levels had risen, her quality of life had improved, and she had resumed activities that had been impossible just a few weeks earlier.

For me, this was a major revelation. I believe that nutritional deficiencies play a far greater role in the fatigue of dialysis patients than most people recognize, and that by correcting these deficiencies, an important difference can be made in patients' lives. Since that experience, I have come across additional energy-enhancing supplements (detailed in this chapter), which you can try to see what works best for you. Just remember to get your doctor's approval before starting your own nutritional supplement regimen.

When people have both health problems, fluid retention and edema can cause unbearable pain. In addition, diabetes can lead to a gastric motility problem called *diabetic gastroparesis (gas-tro-pa-rheeus)*, and dialysis itself can cause a motility problem called *uremic gastropathy*. These disorders, both of which are types of neuropathy, can wreak havoc with blood sugar levels and affect nutrient absorption. Fortunately, alpha-lipoic acid can be helpful in treating all of these forms of neuropathy.

Depending on blood sugar levels—remember that this substance helps control glucose—I generally begin with a dose of 200 to 400 mg of alpha-lipoic acid a day, and then, after a couple of weeks, slowly increase the amount to 600 to 900 mg a day, taken in divided doses on an empty stomach. During that time, if the ALA causes your blood glucose levels to fall too low, you may have to adjust the dose of the supplement or of your diabetes medication.

L-Cysteine and Glutathione

As you learned in Chapter 4 (see page 52), there are many reasons why kidney disease results in anemia (low red blood cell count) and the fatigue that is associated with this disorder. L-cysteine, an amino acid; and glutathione—a potent antioxidant composed of L-cysteine and the amino acids glutamine and glycine—have been found useful not only in helping the body produce energy, but also in aiding the maintenance of red blood cells. Glutathione is one of the most potent antioxidants, and therefore guards red blood cells against the damaging effects of oxidative stress. In fact, I think that low cellular levels of glutathione are an under-reported cause of anemia. I also believe that use of these supplements can reduce the need to prescribe erythropoietin-stimulating agents (ESAs) to increase red blood cell production.

I recommend a formula that combines L-cysteine, glutathione, and vitamin C, or a time-release formula of L-cysteine that prevents levels of glutathione from being depleted. (See pages 180 and 181 of the Resources section.)

SUPPLEMENTS THAT COMBAT INFLAMMATION

As I've mentioned elsewhere in the book, kidney disease, like many other chronic disorders, indicates a state of inflammation. Added to this are the over one hundred inflammation-producing uremic poisons that build up in the bloodstream, and dialysis itself, which can worsen the inflammatory process. This process affects not just the kidneys, but the entire body, including the heart, the liver, and the intestines.

Fortunately, there are several nutritional supplements that can benefit your health by controlling the inflammatory response.

Turmeric

A spice used in cuisines around the world, *turmeric* contains the active ingredient *curcumin,* which has been found to be a potent anti-inflammatory. In India, this spice has long been valued for its medicinal properties.

Scientific studies have found that curcumin inhibits a number of different molecules that are involved in the inflammatory process and has antiviral and antioxidant capabilities. It also has cardiac-protective effects, and, in some of my patients, it appears to help maintain the health of their blood vessels, including that of their fistula or graft.

I recommend taking 200 to 400 mg of turmeric capsules a day. Curcumin has blood-thinning effects, so if you are taking blood thinners such as aspirin, Coumadin (warfarin), or Plavix (clopidogrel), be sure to speak to your doctor before adding this supplement to your regimen.

Quercetin

Quercetin is a *phytochemical* (a plant compound) found in many foods, including apples, berries, cabbage, cauliflower, nuts, and tea. Its powerful anti-inflammatory properties, as well as its anti-allergic properties, are attributed to its strong antioxidant actions. It is also known to work *synergistically* with turmeric, which means that when taken together, these substances produce a beneficial effect that's greater than the sum of their individual actions. Both decrease cardiovascular risk and help restore the health of blood vessels. I recommend using 500 mg of quercetin every day and maintaining that dose throughout treatment.

Omega-3 Fatty Acids

Omega-3 fatty acids, which are found in fatty fish, are known to have strong anti-inflammatory effects as well as being *anti-arrhythmic,* meaning that they prevent abnormal heartbeat rhythms; and *anti-thrombogenic,* meaning that they prevent the formation of dangerous blood clots.

Omega-3 fatty acids are abundant in fish such as mackerel, salmon, herring, lake trout, and sardines. For that reason, depending on your dietary limitations, you should consider adding these fish to your diet. To insure an adequate intake of this nutrient, it is also beneficial to take 1,000 to 2,000 mg of omega-3 fatty acids every day. Because you want your fish oil supplements to be as free as possible from contaminants such as mercury and dioxins, I suggest purchasing them at a health foods store, which is likely to have better-quality supplements. Because omega-3 fish oils can thin the blood, be sure to get your doctor's okay if you are already on a blood thinner such as aspirin, Coumadin (warfarin), or Plavix (clopidogrel).

PROBIOTICS

As first discussed in the section on antibiotics in Chapter 7, *probitoics* are beneficial, or "good," bacteria, most of which live in the digestive system, or gut. These microorganisms help the body digest food, prevent the overgrowth of harmful microorganisms like yeast, and synthesize certain vitamins. A substantial portion of the immune system depends on friendly gut bacteria. Unfortunately, many people—due to poor diet, the use of certain medications, or other factors—have insufficient colonies of these bacteria. Because uremic toxins alter these microorganisms, people with advanced kidney disease can be especially deficient in beneficial bacteria.

Although probiotic supplements are helpful for nearly everyone, and are commonly used to prevent antibiotics from killing off good bacteria during treatment of an infection, these supplements are especially important for someone with kidney failure. You see, the gut can be a resting place for the uremic toxins that accumulate when the kidneys are unable to eliminate them. There, they can perpetuate a host of problems, ranging from inflammation and malnutrition to leaky gut syndrome and yeast infection. Dialysis removes some of these toxins, but it does not remove all. Even in the best case scenario—frequent home HD or daily PD—dialysis doesn't come close to doing the job performed by healthy kidneys. The right probiotics, though, can break down many of the remaining waste products and metabolize them like food so that they can be eliminated through the bowel. This eases the toxic burden on the body. Of course, these supplements also normalize bowel flora and function.

For best results, you'll want to use a kidney-specific probiotic that is designed to work well in the internal environment created by advanced kidney failure and dialysis. I have found that my patients have greater energy and an improved quality of life when they take a probiotic that includes the following strains of bacteria: *S. thermophilus, L. acidophilus,* and *B. longum.* Generally, I recommend starting with one capsule per meal and eventually increasing to two per meal. (Turn to page 180 of the Resources section for further details.)

SUPPLEMENTS THAT SUPPORT BONE HEALTH

As you learned in Chapter 5, to maintain bone health, you have to balance the body's levels of phosphorus, calcium, and parathyroid hormone. Most of the time, physicians focus on these levels and on vitamin D when they address bone support, but I think that more can be done to make sure that your bones remain strong and healthy throughout your treatments. In my practice, I use all of the following nutrients, as warranted, to safeguard the well-being of my patients.

Calcium

In Chapter 4, you learned that your monthly blood work includes a test of your blood calcium levels. A healthy level of calcium is needed to reduce bone loss and decrease the risk of fracture. Calcium also plays an important role in other body functions, such as the control of blood pressure and cholesterol. The goal level of this mineral ranges from 8.4 to 9.5 mg/dL.

As you've read, people on dialysis often have high phosphorus levels and low calcium levels. If your level of calcium is under 8 mg/dL, depending on your phosphorus level, your doctor may prescribe a calcium-based phosphate binder, which will perform the dual role of preventing your body from absorbing excessive amounts of phosphorus and supplementing your calcium. Another option is to take calcium supplements. If your doctor prescribes calcium supplements, be aware that calcium citrate is better absorbed than other forms of this nutrient. To reduce the risk of heavy metal contamination, consider a vegetarian source of calcium or a chelated complex. Remember, too, that calcium can be found naturally in many vegetables that have low or moderate potassium levels, including broccoli, collard greens, kale, and turnip greens. This is the best way to get the calcium you need.

As is true of all nutritional supplements, you should not take calcium supplements unless your doctor prescribes them on the basis of

What Does It Mean
When a Mineral Is Chelated?

When a mineral such as calcium or magnesium is said to be "chelated," it means that the mineral has been combined chemically with amino acids to form a "complex." You may have seen products labeled "chelated calcium" or "chelated magnesium."

Why are minerals chelated? It is thought that chelation makes the mineral more bioavailable—easier for the body to absorb and use.

your blood work. Studies have suggested that too much calcium can increase the risk of heart attack. The goal is not to load up on calcium, but to create the optimal balance of calcium and the other nutrients that your body needs for good bone and heart health. That's why I am not recommending a dosage. Your doctor will prescribe the supplement dose that's right for you.

Magnesium

Like calcium, magnesium is needed to create strong bones, and is also used by the body to regulate blood pressure and perform many other functions. Magnesium is not routinely checked on your monthly labs. When levels of this mineral are tested, doctors look for a normal range of 1.6 to 2.6 mg/dL. This is, of course, *serum magnesium*—in other words, the test measures the magnesium in the blood—but low serum magnesium usually means that levels are low in the cells and bones, as well. When magnesium falls lower than the acceptable range—which most commonly occurs when nutritional status is poor—I normally prescribe a supplement of 200 mg of chelated magnesium per day. I then follow the blood levels closely and increase supplementation slowly until the range of the mineral is acceptable.

Having said that, it's important to explain that people who have advanced kidney disease and are on dialysis tend to have higher-than-normal magnesium levels because their kidneys are no longer able to eliminate the excess. As was the case with calcium, high magnesium—

which is most common when someone is on standard three-times-a-week dialysis—is as dangerous as low magnesium. When magnesium is high, there is no need to take supplements.

Vitamin C

Your bones are composed of hard calcium compounds on a framework of collagen-rich connective tissue. Vitamin C plays a role in the production of collagen as well as the optimal functioning of those cells responsible for making new hard bone. It has also been found that even low (100 mg) doses of vitamin C seem to have an effect on lowering parathyroid hormone (PTH) levels. And as you learned in Chapter 4, for bones to be healthy, PTH levels must be controlled. Vitamin C is also a powerful antioxidant and aids iron absorption and assimilation, so it benefits the person on dialysis in many ways.

Because vitamin C is normally excreted via the kidneys, and therefore can build up in the dialysis patient, I normally recommend 250 mg of vitamin C per day. Note that many brands of renal vitamins contain vitamin C (see page 68 of Chapter 5), so it's important to discuss the need for this nutrient with your physician.

Vitamin D

When a person with normal kidney function obtains vitamin D_3 from the sun or from dietary sources, the vitamin becomes further activated by the kidneys. When someone with advanced kidney disease gets vitamin D from the sun or food, however, this activation doesn't occur. That's why, as described in Chapter 5, people on dialysis are given a vitamin D analogue. This activated form of vitamin D performs the special function of lowering blood levels of parathyroid hormone (PTH), and thus helps prevent the chemical imbalances that can lead to bone loss.

Although you may be getting intravenous or oral doses of vitamin D analogue, I believe that you may still need further vitamin D_3 in the form of a conventional oral supplement. Even without activation by the kidneys, vitamin D_3 contributes to bone health by helping the body better absorb calcium. It also has other beneficial effects, such as strengthening the immune system and aiding the formation of red blood cells.

Several studies have shown that people on dialysis tend to have low levels of vitamin D. Nevertheless, as you may remember from Chapter 4, a test for vitamin D is not a routine part of your blood work, but is usually done on an annual basis unless specified by your doctor. I highly recommend asking your doctor to check your blood level of D and determine if you need supplementation. If your tests show that you are low in vitamin D, I suggest that you start with a relatively small amount—400 to 800 IU of vitamin D_3 daily, taken with food. Because vitamin D can elevate your phosphorus level and can also affect your calcium level, your doctor should take these levels into account before giving the supplements a green light. The goal is to use the least amount of vitamin D possible to prevent or eliminate the deficiency. Follow-up blood tests should be performed on a regular basis to see if the dose should be further increased.

Vitamin K_2

Vitamin K is best known for helping blood to clot, but that benefit is actually true of vitamin K_1—just one form of this powerful nutrient. Another form, K_2, performs other important body functions. First, and most important to our discussion of bone health, vitamin K_2 guides calcium into the bones and prevents it from being leached out. This is why low levels of vitamin K are associated with fractures and poor bone density. And by keeping calcium in the bones, where it belongs, vitamin K_2 also protects blood vessels. You see, when calcium levels are low, as they often are when someone is on dialysis, the body tries to get the calcium it needs by leaching it out of the bones. Once the calcium makes its way into the blood, it is deposited on the blood vessels and other tissues. This can lead to serious problems, including *aortic stenosis*, a narrowing of the valve between the left ventricle of the heart and the aorta. So by preventing calcium from moving from the bones to the bloodstream, K_2 not only protects bone health but also helps prevent vascular calcification. This is important for dialysis patients, for whom this disorder can run rampant.

I recommend this supplement if you have elevated levels of parathyroid hormone (PTH), which can compromise bone health. I usually start with a dose of 40 mcg of vitamin K_2 a day, and slowly increase to 80 mcg. If you are taking the blood thinner Coumadin (warfarin), you should not take vitamin K in any form as it can decrease the effectiveness of the medication.

Bone Mineral Supplements

As you have seen, calcium, magnesium, vitamin D_3, vitamin K_2, and vitamin C all are important for bone health. Beyond this, several trace minerals that we have not yet discussed are also essential. They do not need to be supplemented in large quantities, but deficiencies of these minerals can definitely affect the well-being of your bones. They include boron, copper, manganese, and zinc. These, as well as other nutrients

Endothelial Cell Dysfunction and Dialysis

The *endothelial cells* make up the layer of cells that line the interior of the blood vessels. When these cells function properly, they regulate a number of vital processes, including dilation (widening) and constriction (narrowing) of the blood vessels, control of the volume of fluids that pass from the blood into the tissues, control of blood clotting, and much more. When endothelial cells are not able to function as they should, one result is that the arteries stiffen and become less elastic. This means that the heart must exert more effort to eject blood into the arteries, placing an ever-increasing burden on the heart and leading to high blood pressure. Endothelial dysfunction also makes it difficult for the heart to relax. All of this raises the risk of heart attack and stroke.

Hypertension and diabetes—both of which are common in dialysis patients—can contribute to endothelial dysfunction. Dialysis itself also appears to contribute to endothelial dysfunction and the resulting heart-related complications, with people on hemodialysis experiencing more endothelial problems than those on peritoneal dialysis.

The bottom line is if you are on dialysis—and especially if you are on hemodialysis and/or also have diabetes—you have to do your best to treat endothelial dysfunction. Turn to page 114 to read about the supplements that can be used to help prevent and control this disorder.

vital to bone health, are often combined in comprehensive bone-health supplements.

Combination bone mineral supplements have pros and cons. On one hand, most people who are on dialysis take a lot of pills, so it can make sense to use a supplement that offers several nutrients in a single dose. On the other hand, if you take renal vitamins, you may already be getting enough zinc, which is a common ingredient of bone supplements. Remember, too, that bone supplements usually contain potassium and magnesium—minerals that must be monitored in people on dialysis. That's why it's so important to speak to your doctor before using a bone mineral supplement.

SUPPLEMENTS TO TREAT ENDOTHELIAL DYSFUNCTION

Endothelial dysfunction, a disorder of the cells that line the blood vessels, is all too common in the dialysis population. (See the inset on page 113 to learn more.) It can raise blood pressure and make it difficult for the heart to do its job, increasing the risk of heart attack and stroke.

What can you do to treat this problem? First, if you have diabetes, do your best to keep your blood sugar under control. Uncontrolled blood sugars can greatly contribute to inflammation and endothelial problems, so it's important to regulate your diet, use your diabetes medications as directed, and include exercise in your daily regimen as much as possible.

Also make use of supplements that can improve the environment of blood vessels and, as a result, enhance endothelial health. Coenzyme Q_{10} (discussed on page 102), magnesium (page 110), turmeric (page 106), quercetin (page 107), and vitamin K_2 (page 112), can all be helpful in this respect. In addition, consider using the three supplements that are discussed below.

Resveratrol

A powerful antioxidant and anti-inflammatory, *resveratrol* is produced by several plants but is best known as the active ingredient in red wine. Resveratrol enhances the actions of nitric oxide (NO), which relaxes blood vessel walls, allowing blood to flow easily. It has been shown to help restore endothelial function and maintain healthy heart function.

I believe that everyone with kidney disease—and, therefore, everyone on dialysis—should take resveratrol because it can help maintain and improve the health of blood vessels, and may even aid in keeping fistulas and grafts open and functioning. Because it is a blood thinner, though, it should not be taken without the approval of your nephrologist, especially if you are using any other blood thinners like aspirin, Coumadin (warfarin), or Plavix (clopidogrel).

I generally start my patients on 50 mg per day. If the supplement is well tolerated, which it usually is, I gradually increase the dose to 100 mg per day.

Garlic

The important role that garlic can play in heart health has been well documented. Garlic appears to boost the body's production of hydrogen sulfide (H_2S), which relaxes blood vessels, promoting blood flow. Garlic has also been shown to decrease cholesterol and prevent the formation of plaque on artery walls, all of which adds up to a stronger cardiovascular system.

Garlic can be administered in several ways, but when someone is on dialysis, it's important to know exactly how much is being taken. That's why I recommend starting with a 200 mg capsule of aged garlic extract and increasing slowly to 400 mg per day. If you are on a blood thinner like aspirin, Coumadin (warfarin), or Plavix (clopidogrel), speak to your doctor before taking garlic supplements, as they can increase the chance of bruising and bleeding.

Pomegranate

Pomegranate juice is one of nature's most concentrated sources of antioxidants and provides powerful cardiovascular protection by restoring endothelial health. Specifically, it augments nitric oxide, which signals the muscles of the blood vessels to relax, thereby increasing blood flow through the arteries and veins. Nitric oxide also reduces injury to the blood vessels, helping prevent the development of atherosclerosis. A study of one hundred dialysis patients found that patients taking pomegranate juice had less atherosclerosis, as well as lower blood pressure and better cholesterol profiles. Pomegranate has actually been found to have some of the blood pressure-lowering effects of ACE inhibitors, but without the side effects normally associated with these drugs.

You can either drink pomegranate juice or take pomegranate extract supplements. If you choose the juice, I recommend consuming three to four ounces a day. If you prefer to take capsules, I recommend a dose of 250 to 500 mg daily.

PROTEIN SUPPLEMENTS

People on dialysis have an unusually high need for protein. Because some protein is lost in the process of dialysis, and dialysis impairs the body's use and processing of the amino acids that make up protein, you can actually become malnourished if you don't get all the protein you need.

Chapter 9 will fill you in on the high-quality proteins you should include in your dialysis diet (see page 122), but unfortunately, even the most carefully planned menus may not always provide as much of this nutrient as you require. If the albumin level in your monthly blood work shows that you are not getting enough protein (see page 57 of Chapter 4), your dietitian or nephrologist may recommend a protein powder, which is a concentrated source of high-quality protein. Most dietitians prescribe one of several standard protein supplements, and for many people, these are excellent choices. But in my experience, I've found that sometimes a different protein powder is needed—one that can positively change the body's chemistry and help rebuild it. This requires some clarification.

Throughout this book, I explain that kidney disease in and of itself indicates an inflammatory process, and that the process of dialysis, while lifesaving, increases total body inflammation. In fact, dialysis places great stress on the body, actually causing it to break down its protein stores. This state of "breaking down" is called a *catabolic state*. When your body is catabolic, even if you provide it with a supply of protein in the form of food or a supplement powder, it may not be able to use it properly. This is why when a patient is not doing well on the protein powder she's been using, and especially if she shows marked signs of inflammation, I often suggest a protein supplement that can change her body chemistry to an *anabolic state*—a state in which organs and tissues are built up rather than being broken down. These specialized protein powders supply potent antioxidants; omega-3 fatty acids; and amino acids, including *leucine*—an essential amino acid that has been shown to not only help prevent muscle loss, but also stimulate the building of muscles and other tissues. These supplements can be used in addition to or instead of the one you may already be taking. Just be sure to get your doctor's and dietitian's approval if you think that a different powder might be a good option. (Turn to page 181 of the Resources section to learn more about these specialized supplements.)

How much protein powder should you take? Usually, it's appropriate to take a tablespoon once or twice a day, depending on your nutritional status. If your monthly tests show a need for supplemental protein, work with your renal dietitian to come up with a regimen that will meet your specific dietary needs. It can make a positive difference in the way you feel.

IN CONCLUSION

The successful treatment of kidney failure involves much more than dialysis. It also means carefully monitoring your diet and taking supplements that will help compensate for the loss of kidney function, offset some of the adverse effects of dialysis, enhance energy, combat inflammation, maintain gut health, protect bone health, and support cardiovascular function.

In my practice, I have seen just how effective the right supplements can be. They can vastly improve a patient's health and enrich her quality of life. However, I cannot overemphasize the fact that before you introduce any new supplements to your regimen, you *must* discuss them with your nephrologist, who—based on your blood work, your current meds, and other factors—can best determine whether these nutrients are right for you.

9

*E*ating Right on Dialysis

When you're on dialysis, you need the same nutrients that a person with healthy kidneys requires. Protein, carbohydrates, fat, water, vitamins, and minerals are all necessary if the body is to create energy and carry on its many functions, including the repair of tissues and organs. But because your kidneys cannot filter out toxins, limitations have to be placed on those substances that can build up in your bloodstream and make you sick. Dialysis does remove some potentially harmful substances from the body, but it does not eliminate wastes as completely as functioning kidneys would. Moreover, between treatments, both toxins and fluids can build up. That's why a healthy dialysis diet limits foods that are more likely to produce toxic wastes, and also limits water and other fluids that can accumulate.

It's important to understand that the needs of someone on dialysis differ from those of someone who has chronic kidney disease but is not on dialysis, so if you've been on a CKD diet and are just starting dialysis, you will have to make some changes. The biggest change will be that you can now have more protein—a nutrient that's limited when someone has CKD but is not being dialyzed. Your diet will also greatly depend on the type of dialysis you are having. If you have read the earlier chapters in this book, you'll understand why. Standard in-center hemodialysis takes place three times a week for just a few hours per session. Because this can allow a significant buildup of fluids and toxins between treatments, people on standard hemodialysis have to very carefully limit their intake of fluids and certain foods. Nocturnal hemodialysis and home hemodialysis are performed for more hours a week, and peritoneal dialysis is used every single day, allowing more dietary freedom. In general, the more frequent the dialysis, the more liberal the diet. But perhaps the most important "rule" is that every person on dialysis is unique. This chapter is designed to guide your choices and help you eat as healthfully as possible, but it's essential that you work with your dietitian, who—based on your blood work, your weight, your medications, and other factors—will create a menu plan that is tailored to your specific needs.

SHOOTING FOR THE OPTIMAL DIET

No one can dispute the fact that being on a dialysis-based diet is difficult. First of all, there are a lot of restrictions. Second, a loss of appetite, which is common in people on dialysis, can complicate your efforts to eat well. Despite that, it's important to aim for the best nutrition possible because food is your most important medicine. If you stick to a good diet, you will not only help your body better perform all the functions necessary for life, but you will also control the buildup of toxins and fluids between dialysis treatments, help control the inflammation that is part of kidney disease, and improve your overall health.

What is the ideal dialysis diet? First, it is high enough in protein to meet the dialysis patient's higher-than-normal needs for this nutrient. (You'll learn about this later in the chapter.) It is also high in anti-inflammatory fruits and veggies. And it provides antioxidants while limiting the amounts of sodium, phosphorus, and potassium.

The following pages discuss the key nutrients that most people on dialysis have to monitor, but never forget that you should always follow the *specific* advice provided by your healthcare team. Also work with your dietitian to determine the best timing of your meals, especially on dialysis days. This is particularly important if you have diabetes or if your blood pressure tends to fall too low during dialysis treatments. For detailed nutritional information about specific foods, be sure to check out the websites Self Nutrition Data and Nephron Information Center Food Values (see page 179 of the Resources section), both of which have great "Search" features.

Protein

When you had earlier-stage kidney disease and were not yet on dialysis, your doctor may have told you to lower your consumption of protein because your kidneys were not able to handle large amounts of this nutrient. Without normal filtration through the kidneys, a diet high in protein would have resulted in the accumulation of dangerous waste products in your blood. But, as I mentioned earlier, once you start dialysis, you usually have to *increase* your consumption of proteins. It's important to understand why.

You may already know that protein plays an important role in the body by providing the amino acids that are required to build muscle and maintain healthy cells, organs, and bones. You may not know, though, that someone on dialysis requires more protein than the average adult for two reasons: because some protein is lost in the process of dialysis, and because dialysis impairs the body's ability to use and process amino acids. In fact, dialysis patients who don't get enough protein can develop a disorder called *protein-energy malnutrition (PEM)*.

Most people on dialysis are encouraged to eat as much high-quality proteins as they can. The average patient needs about 1.2 grams of protein per kilogram of body weight per day. This means that every day, a 70-kilogram (150-pound) male would need to eat about 84 grams of protein (70 x 1.2 = 84)—the equivalent of roughly 12 ounces of cooked chicken.

Although protein consumption is a must, when you're on dialysis, some proteins are better than others. Remember that waste products do accumulate between dialysis sessions and that your treatments can't filter out all the toxins in your blood. That's why you have to focus on proteins that provide you with all the amino acids you need, but that produce relatively low amounts of waste. Specifically, you must avoid foods that are higher in phosphorus. On page 122, you'll find a list of high-quality proteins as well as a list of proteins whose consumption should be restricted. As always, leaner, lower-fat selections are best for total health, and the meat should not be processed, because almost all processed foods provide too much sodium, are "enhanced" with phosphorus, and are pro-inflammatory. If at all possible, choose grass-fed meats. Although soy products such as tofu and soy milk are great sources of protein, restrict yourself to one serving a day because many soy-based foods are high in potassium.

The Best Proteins on Dialysis

- Egg whites
- Fish
- Meat, such as lean beef and pork
- Poultry, such as chicken and turkey breast
- Soy products, such as tofu and soy milk

Proteins That Should Be Limited on Dialysis

- Milk, cheese, yogurt, and other dairy products
- Processed meats

If the albumin levels on your monthly blood work are too low, indicating that you may not be eating enough protein or enough calories, your dietitian may suggest that you take a protein supplement. (To learn more about albumin levels, see page 57 of Chapter 4. To learn more about protein powders, see page 116 of Chapter 8.)

Sodium

In Chapter 6, you learned that people on dialysis have to watch their sodium levels as a means of limiting fluid gains and controlling blood pressure. In general, you should restrict your sodium to 1,500 to 2,000 mg a day, depending on your physical condition and the type of dialysis you are using. (See page 82 for more about sodium restrictions and to learn the difference between sodium and salt.) Clearly, you should limit your use of table salt, which is the number-one source of sodium for most people. But you also have to be aware of many other common high-sodium foods, including the following:

- Baking soda and baking powder
- Canned and dehydrated soups, broths, and gravies
- Canned vegetables
- Cheese
- Cured meats, such as bacon and salami, and processed deli meats, such as turkey

- Frozen dinners
- Marmite yeast extract
- Pickled foods such as olives and dill pickles
- Powdered broths and bouillon cubes
- Saltwater crab
- Snack foods such as pretzels, cheese puffs, and potato chips
- Soy sauce and tamari

One factor that most, though not all, of the above foods have in common is that they are processed. As already mentioned, a large amount of salt is used in almost all processed and prepared foods. You can eliminate a good amount of sodium by avoiding processed foods and, instead, basing your diet on fresh fruits, vegetables, and meats, and seasoning your dishes without salt or salty flavorings. When you do choose to use commercial products, look for lower-sodium or no-salt-added versions. For instance, one popular chicken noodle soup contains 790 mg of sodium per 1-cup serving. If your limit is 1,500 mg per day, that cup will use up about half of your daily allotment. If you choose a lower-sodium version of the same soup, you'll get 410 mg per cup. That is still a lot of sodium in one shot, but if you really want canned soup, it's a better choice.

Fortunately, all packaged foods have Nutrition Facts labels that tell you exactly how much sodium there is per serving so that you can make informed choices. When reading these nutrition labels, be sure to pay attention to portion size. Going back to the example of the low-sodium soup, you would probably be able to work a one-cup serving into your daily meal plan, but the full can—which includes two portions—would make it very difficult to stay within your sodium limits. (See the inset on page 124 to learn how to get the information you need from a food label.)

Potassium

The mineral potassium is necessary to keep the heart, muscles, and nerves working properly. But you can have too much potassium, and when the kidneys fail, the body loses its ability to eliminate excess amounts from the system. When this happens, potassium can build up

How to Read a Food Label
Tips for People with Chronic Kidney Disease (CKD)

If you have CKD, you may need to limit some nutrients in your diet such as sodium, phosphorus, or potassium. You should limit saturated and trans fats, too. Read the food label to help make healthy food choices for your kidneys.

- Check the Nutrition Facts label for sodium.

- Check the ingredient list for added phosphorus and potassium.

- Look for claims on the label, like "low saturated fat" or "sodium free."

What Should I Look for on the Nutrition Facts Label?

Look for **sodium** on the Nutrition Facts label. Some Nutrition Facts labels will list **phosphorus** and **potassium**, too, but they do not have to.

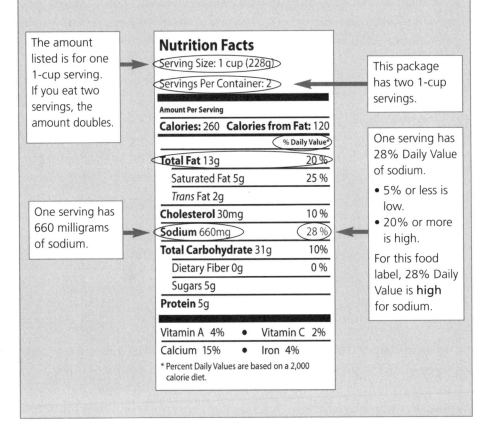

The amount listed is for one 1-cup serving. If you eat two servings, the amount doubles.

This package has two 1-cup servings.

One serving has 660 milligrams of sodium.

One serving has 28% Daily Value of sodium.
- 5% or less is low.
- 20% or more is high.

For this food label, 28% Daily Value is **high** for sodium.

Nutrition Facts
Serving Size: 1 cup (228g)
Servings Per Container: 2

Amount Per Serving

Calories: 260 **Calories from Fat:** 120

	% Daily Value*
Total Fat 13g	20 %
Saturated Fat 5g	25 %
Trans Fat 2g	
Cholesterol 30mg	10 %
Sodium 660mg	28 %
Total Carbohydrate 31g	10%
Dietary Fiber 0g	0 %
Sugars 5g	
Protein 5g	

Vitamin A 4%	•	Vitamin C 2%
Calcium 15%	•	Iron 4%

* Percent Daily Values are based on a 2,000 calorie diet.

What Should I Look for on the Ingredient List?

1. Look for **phosphorus**, or for words with PHOS, on the ingredient list. Many packaged foods have phosphorus. Choose a different food when the ingredient list has PHOS on the label.

> **Ingredients:** Rehydrated potatoes (Water, Potatoes, Sodium acid pyro**phos**phate), Beef (Beef, Water, Salt, Sodium **phos**phate), Wine . . .
>
> *This ingredient list shows that the food has added phosphorus.*

2. Look for **potassium** on the ingredient list. For example, potassium chloride can be used in place of salt in some packaged foods, like canned soups and tomato products. Limit foods with potassium on the ingredient list.

> **Ingredients:** Tomato juice, Vegetable juice blend, **Potassium** chloride, Sugar, Magnesium, Salt, Vitamin C (Ascorbic acid), Citric acid, Spice extract, Flavoring, Disodium inosinate, Disodium guanylate.
>
> *This ingredient list shows that the food has added potassium.*

Did You Know?
Ingredients are listed in order of the amount in the food. The food has the most of the first ingredient on the list, and the least of the last ingredient on the list.

Look for Claims on Food Packages to Help You Find Foods:

Lower in Saturated/Trans Fat	Lower in Sodium*
• Saturated fat free	• Sodium free
• Low saturated fat	• Very low sodium
• Less saturated fat	• Low sodium
• Trans fat free	• Reduced salt

* Reprinted courtesy of the National Kidney Disease Education Program of the National Institutes of Health (visit www.nkdep.nih.gov).

to the point where it causes a host of problems, including heart failure. Dialysis does remove some potassium from the system, but it does not remove all, and, of course, this mineral accumulates in the blood between treatments. This is a bigger problem for standard in-center hemodialysis patients, because the dialysis sessions are short and take place just three times a week. People on nocturnal HD have normal to high levels. The longer hours of treatment remove a good deal of the potassium, but since these people tend to feel better, they actually eat more—including more potassium. People on peritoneal dialysis tend to have lower potassium levels.

Because dialysis can eliminate only so much potassium from your body, you have to do your part to keep your intake of this substance down. In general, people on hemodialysis have to limit their daily intake of potassium to 2,000 to 3,000 mg, and people on peritoneal dialysis can have between 3,000 and 4,000 mg a day. But, as always, your dietitian will determine your personal potassium allowance based on your blood work.

Restricting potassium means choosing your foods carefully. Nearly all foods contain some potassium, but some are higher in this substance than others. When selecting foods, try to focus on those with a relatively low level—foods like apples and cucumbers—and avoid or limit foods that have higher levels—bananas and potatoes, for instance. Remember, too, that serving size is very important. (As a rule, aim for a half-cup portion.) A large amount of even a low-potassium food can provide you with too much of this mineral. Unfortunately, potassium is usually not included on the Nutrition Facts labels found on most packaged foods. (Some companies do list potassium, but they are not required to do so.) But the ingredients list does have to include products such as *"potassium* chloride" if they're used in the food. So while you're checking the sodium content, be sure to read through the ingredients list, as well, and avoid or limit foods whose ingredients include the word *"potassium."*

The following lists highlight some of the best and the worst foods in regard to potassium content. You'll find more complete lists by checking some of the informational websites listed in the Resources section, which begins on page 177. Your renal dietitian can also steer you toward low-postassium foods and products.

Low-Potassium Fruits, Vegetables, and Other Foods

- Apples
- Asparagus
- Berries
- Bread (not whole grain)
- Broccoli
- Cauliflower
- Cherries
- Corn
- Cranberries
- Cucumbers
- Garlic
- Grapes
- Green beans
- Lettuce
- Mushrooms
- Onions
- Pasta and noodles (not whole grain)
- Peaches
- Peppers
- Pineapple
- Plums
- Tangerines
- White rice
- Yellow summer squash
- Zucchini squash

High-Potassium Fruits, Vegetables, and Other Foods

- Acorn squash
- Apricots
- Avocados
- Bananas
- Beets
- Brussels sprouts
- Carrots and carrot juice
- Clams
- Dates
- Figs
- Kiwi
- Lima beans
- Melons
- Milk, cheese, yogurt, and other dairy products
- Nectarines
- Nuts
- Oranges and orange juice
- Prunes and prune juice
- Raisins
- Rutabagas
- Salt substitutes that contain potassium
- Sardines
- Spinach
- Sweet potatoes (especially baked)
- Tomatoes and tomato juice
- White potatoes (especially baked)
- Winter squash

A final word about potassium: You can actually leach or "dialyze" some of this mineral out of certain vegetables. This can make it possible to include slightly larger portions of these foods in your diet. See the inset below for step-by-step instructions on leaching potassium out of frozen greens, potatoes, and several other common veggies.

Leaching the Potassium Out of Vegetables

If you've looked at the lists on page 127, you know that some vegetables are higher in potassium than others. Fortunately, a process called *leaching* can remove some (but not all) of the potassium found in some vegetables. Usually, you can have a half-cup of foods that are low or moderately high in potassium. If you leach out some of this mineral, you can eat a little more, although you still have to control portion size. Be sure to ask your dietitian about the amount of leached vegetables that can be worked into your meal plan. The following directions will help you remove potassium from white potatoes, sweet potatoes, beets, carrots, rutabagas, cauliflower, mushrooms, squash, and frozen greens.

1. If you're using root vegetables, peel them and slice them 1/8-inch thick. If you're using cauliflower or squash, cut the vegetable into small pieces. If you're using a package of frozen vegetables, thaw them and be sure to drain off any liquid. Then rinse the vegetables in warm water for a few seconds.

2. Place the vegetables in a large bowl or pot and fill it with warm water, using ten times the amount of water as the amount of vegetables. (For example, if you have a cup of diced potatoes, use ten cups of warm water.) Soak for a minimum of two hours. If you decide to soak the veggies for a longer period of time, change the water every four hours or so.

3. Drain off the soaking water and again rinse the vegetables in warm water for a few seconds.

4. Cook the vegetables in five times the amount of water as the amount of vegetables.

Phosphorus

Phosphorus is necessary for health. But without functioning kidneys to remove excess amounts, this nutrient can accumulate in the blood and affect both bone and heart health. Dialysis removes some of the excess phosphorus from the blood, but it can't filter out all of it. That's why your phosphorus levels are tested every month and why your dietitian probably recommends limiting high-phosphorus foods. This substance is a problem regardless of the mode of dialysis that's being used.

Phosphorus is found in all foods, but a number of foods are relatively high in this substance and should be avoided entirely or consumed in very limited amounts. Many of these foods are listed below. Phosphorus, like potassium, is usually not included on the Nutrition Facts labels found on packaged foods, but the ingredients lists have to include substances such as "sodium acid pyro*phos*phate," "sodium *phos*phate," and "*phos*phoric acid" if they're used in the food. Look for ingredients that include "*phos*"—an indication that the product contains added phosphorus.

High-Phosphorus Foods and Beverages

- Beer and ale
- Bran cereals
- Brewer's yeast
- Canned iced tea
- Caramels
- Carp
- Chocolate drinks
- Crayfish
- Dark colas and some other sodas (check the ingredients lists)
- Dried peas and beans, including baked beans, kidney beans, etc.
- Meats that have been "enhanced" (injected with a solution of water and other ingredients)
- Milk, cheese, yogurt, and other dairy products
- Nuts
- Organ meats such as liver
- Oysters
- Sardines
- Seeds
- Wheat germ
- Whole grains and whole grain products

Your doctor may order phosphate binders that will help control the amount of phosphorus that your body absorbs from foods and beverages. These medications are discussed in greater detail on page 69 of Chapter 5.

Fluids

No chapter on dialysis nutrition would be complete without a mention of fluids because fluid restriction is so important—especially if you're on standard in-center hemodialysis, which can allow fluids to build up between treatments. If you have not already read the section "Keeping

---

Following the Dialysis Diet When You're Dining Out

By now, you're aware of the many restrictions imposed by your dialysis diet. Do these "food rules" mean that you have to eat all your meals at home so you can have complete control of your diet? Fortunately, the answer is *no*. You can still enjoy eating out with friends and family as long as you choose both the restaurant and the foods very carefully.

Some restaurants pre-season or pre-marinate many of their foods, so the first thing you'll want to do is find an establishment that starts with plain, unseasoned foods that can be prepared to order, without salt and high-sodium ingredients like marinades and sauces. Once you've found an accommodating restaurant, the following tips should help you stick to your diet:

- If you're going to dine out later in the day, cut back on fluids and high-potassium foods during the day. This will give you a little more leeway—and a greater margin for error—when you're at the restaurant.

- For breakfast, consider an egg white omelet with low-potassium vegetables such as onion and green bell pepper. To avoid high-sodium, -potassium, -and -phosphorus foods, skip add-ins and sides like cheese, avocado, sausage, ham, and bacon. Other than egg whites, good breakfast options include pineapple; puffed rice cereal with rice milk; and toasted white or sourdough breads, English muffins, and

the Right Fluid Balance" in Chapter 6 (see page 78), please go back and read it now. It provides important information about how much liquid you should drink and which beverages can best contribute to your over-all health. The bottom line is that to avoid blood pressure highs and lows as well as serious heart problems, you must speak to your nutritionist about your fluid limits and do your best to remain within them.

THE IMPORTANCE OF FRUITS AND VEGGIES

Everyone tells you that a diet high in fruits and vegetables is beneficial, and it's just as true for people on dialysis as it is for people with fully

bagels. (Avoid whole grain products except in very small quantities.) Instead of orange juice, try cranberry or apple juice.

- At lunch and breakfast, ask for a 3- to 4-ounce portion of grilled, baked, or broiled steak, burgers, poultry, pork chops, or seafood. Dialysis-friendly side dishes include a small green salad with a simple oil-and-vinegar dressing; steamed rice; noodles or pasta; or vegeta-bles such as summer squash, corn, or green beans. Remember to limit your portions.

- When you place your order, be sure to request that your meal be pre-pared without salt, onion or garlic salt, salted butter, soy sauce, pick-les, capers, or any other seasoning or condiment that's high in sodium. If your food tastes salty, stop eating it and ask for something else. Make it clear that you will get seriously ill if the foods are not pre-pared as you request.

- For dessert, request berries, sherbet, angel food cake, or pound cake. Avoid chocolate and anything that's dairy-based, including puddings, custards, and cheesecake.

- If your doctor has prescribed phosphorus binders, make sure to carry the bottle with you and to take them exactly as directed—before, dur-ing, or right after the meal, as the case may be. Since you can't be sure of how much phosphorus is being provided by the food you're served in a restaurant, phosphorus binders are essential when dining out.

What Is Considered a Fluid?

While you probably realize that all beverages—water, juice, coffee, etc.—are fluids, you may be surprised to learn that any food that melts at room temperature also belongs in this category. All of the following are considered fluids:

- Ice
- Ice cream
- Italian ices
- Jell-O gelatin dessert
- Popsicles
- Sherbet and sorbet
- Soup

In addition, many fruits and vegetables contain a lot of water that adds to your fluid intake. Produce with a relatively high water content includes apples, cantaloupe, celery, grapes, lettuce, melons, oranges, tomatoes, and watermelon. An apple can be about 85 percent water; lettuce, over 90 percent. How can you figure this into your fluid intake? As a rule of thumb, for every 4 ounces (half cup) of vegetables or fruit you eat, make an assumption that about 75 percent—3 ounces, in other words—is fluid.

functioning kidneys. In fact, it may be *more* important for someone on dialysis. Let's look at the most important benefits that the right produce has to offers.

In Chapter 1, you learned that healthy kidneys help control the body's acid-base balance, and that when the kidneys fail to function, the bloodstream becomes too acidic. This is dangerous because acidity promotes inflammation and malnutrition, both of which are rampant in the dialysis population. Although dialysis treatments, which use an alkalyzing "bicarbonate bath," help lower acidity, without dietary adjustments, many people still don't have a healthy pH. And the standard American diet—high in meat, poultry, fish, and cheese—only contributes to the acidity. How can you help restore balance? Many fruits and vegetables actually have the effect of alkalizing the body. Some especially good choices include apples, berries, broccoli, cherries, lettuce, onions, peppers, and pineapple. These foods, along with mildly alkaline water (see page 83), can do a lot to eliminate acidity and promote healing.

Fruits and vegetables are also rich in antioxidants such as vitamins A, C, and E. These substances are important because they combat the free radical damage that plays a major role in the development of common disorders such as heart disease, diabetes, and cancer. Although all fruits and vegetables contain some antioxidants, those richest in these health-promoting substances include deeply pigmented fruits such as blackberries, blueberries, cherries, and cranberries; and vegetables such as asparagus, broccoli, and corn.

It should go without saying that you must choose those vegetables and fruits that allow you to stay within your specific dietary limitations. In most cases, that means selecting produce that is low in potassium (see page 127 of this chapter) and also preparing your veggies without salt and high-sodium flavorings. If you have diabetes, you should also avoid foods that have a high glycemic index (GI), as foods with a high GI break down quickly during digestion, releasing glucose into your bloodstream. Your nutritionist can guide you to foods that have a lower GI.

SAMPLE MENU CHOICES

You now know a lot about the foods that are the best choices on dialysis, as well as the foods that should be avoided or eaten in very limited quantities. Believe me, I know that it's a lot to learn, and it may seem that all your favorite meals are no-nos. Let me assure you that by making some simple substitutions, you can eat well and help maximize your overall health. Below, I've suggested a few options for each meal of the day. Show these meal ideas to your dietitian to see if they're right for you, and ask him to come up with additional menus that suit both your dietary needs and your tastes.

Good Breakfast Choices

- A bowl of rice-based cereal such as puffed rice, topped with rice milk or soy milk and some antioxidant-packed fruit such as blueberries, strawberries, or cherries.

- Scrambled egg whites or an egg white omelet that includes low-potassium veggies such as broccoli, onions, and peppers.

Good Lunch Choices

- A salad of iceberg lettuce and a little romaine, mixed with low-potassium vegetables such as cucumbers and peppers and a dressing of oil and balsamic vinegar. For protein, top the salad with a little grilled chicken breast (3 to 4 ounces).

- A sandwich of whole wheat pita and 3 to 4 ounces of grilled chicken breast or canned tuna without mayonnaise. Although whole wheat bread tends to be high in potassium, a whole wheat pita keeps the potassium under control and is higher in nutrients than white bread.

Good Dinner Choices

- A small portion of fish (3 or 4 ounces), with a side dish of steamed asparagus, green beans, or broccoli. Sprinkle on a little lemon juice for flavor.

- A small portion (½ cup) of cooked quinoa (*keen-wa*) tossed with a little olive oil, sautéed garlic, and sliced steamed zucchini. If you like pasta, a healthier substitute is 4 ounces of cooked spaghetti squash tossed with a little olive oil and garlic.

IN CONCLUSION

Good nutrition is important for everyone, and it is essential when you're on dialysis. Look at what you eat as more than just food. View it as a means of making yourself better. There are many nutritional changes that you will have to get used to—some difficult, some not so difficult. To approach them in the most positive way possible, look for healthy substitutions for the foods you're used to eating and ask your dietitian to create a menu that defines what you *can* eat, not what you can't eat.

10

Keeping Your Mind, Body, and Spirit in the Game

ialysis is hard. It means a big change in your life—not just because of the treatments, but also because of dietary restrictions, medication regimens, and side effects such as fatigue. Yet I know many people who have experienced years of chronic illness, including dialysis, and have been able to keep their mind and spirit "in the game." Instead of letting their medical situation rule their lives and dim their view of the future, they have done their best to develop a positive attitude and make changes that promote not just better physical health, but also mental and spiritual soundness. It's not easy, but it can be done. In this chapter, I offer some ways in which you can strengthen your mind, body, and spirit and learn to thrive on dialysis.

GETTING YOUR MIND IN THE GAME

When people are told that they need dialysis, they usually experience strong emotions, including fear of the unknown ("What's going to happen to me?"), anger, ("Why me?"), and loss of control ("Will I be able to take care of myself? Will I be a burden to my family?"). These emotions can be disabling and prevent you from getting your mind in the game.

Before you can take charge of your life and move toward greater wellness, you have to get past your initial emotions and accept that your life has changed. Generally, there are three steps involved in this process.

135

Step 1: Acceptance

The people who do best on dialysis are those who accept it. They need to, because starting treatment means a lot of changes and a huge learning curve. Note that acceptance does *not* mean giving up; rather, it means saying, "I accept the fact that this has happened, and I want to do everything I can to improve my life and the lives of those around me."

People who are in denial do not do well. They refuse to change their diet and their lifestyle, and they may miss dialysis sessions. Over time, they often make themselves sicker, so that a vicious cycle develops. The less they do to care for themselves, the worse they feel, which makes them even less able and willing to follow a healthy diet and go for treatment. Refusal to accept the need for dialysis and other changes means more than a "bad attitude." It is the difference between getting better and getting progressively more ill.

Step 2: Adaptation

Once you accept the need for dialysis, you can adapt your thinking to the changes that are taking place in your life and begin to form a new life plan for making the best of your situation. If, for example, you have begun dialysis in a dedicated center, you may start thinking about other dialysis options, perhaps home hemodialysis or peritoneal dialysis. If in-center dialysis is your only option, you may start looking for ways to make your sessions better.

When I was very young, for a brief time, I studied martial arts. Although I had two left feet, in addition to discovering the importance of proper breathing (discussed later in the chapter), I also learned the following invaluable mantra, "If you can conceive and believe, then you can achieve." The beginning of positive change is conceiving of that change. Once you believe in yourself, you'll be amazed by what you can achieve.

Step 3: Action, Not Reaction

After acceptance and adaptation comes action. You have accepted the need for change, and you have adapted your thinking to this new reality. Now it's time to take action. No longer will you simply react to what is going on around you. You are ready to take charge of your health and your life.

KEEPING YOUR MIND IN THE GAME

Some people do their best to take a positive approach to dialysis but find it difficult to maintain a "strong mind" over time. The day-to-day efforts

Being Informed Can Be the Best Medicine

One of the best ways to deal with your fears of dialysis is to learn all that you can about kidney failure, dialysis options, diet, medication, nutritional supplements, and other aspects of treatment. People who become informed usually experience less fear of the unknown and a greater sense of control. Studies show that they also report fewer symptoms and have more confidence in their ability to manage those problems that they do have. Naturally, the information they gather permits them to make decisions that can contribute to better health and a much more satisfying life.

Picking up this book was a good first step in your journey to become well-informed. Within these pages, you'll learn a lot of what you want to know. But be sure to take advantage of *all* the resources that are available to you. When you get your blood work, read it and discuss it with your dialysis team so that you fully understand how your body is responding to your dialysis and medications. Speak to your dietitian about menus and recipes that can help you feel your best. Check the websites listed in the Resources section in the back of this book (see page 177). Many of them offer a wealth of information, suggestions, and guidelines, as well as links to other great Internet sites. Also contact your local medical or dialysis center to see if it offers education classes on various aspects of chronic kidney disease and dialysis. These resources can enable you to make good decisions regarding treatment, find solutions to problems as they crop up, and maintain a positive, proactive approach to your healthcare.

needed to manage all the different aspects of care, plus the physical effects of kidney failure and dialysis, can certainly chip away at your resolve. How can you avoid being worn down mentally by your health-care routine?

Developing a healthy mindset does not occur overnight. The key is to "practice" each day until it becomes an integral part of your life. How can you practice a healthy mindset? One great way is to use positive affirmation to "re-set" your thinking. Every morning when you awaken, look in the mirror and say, "Today is going to be a great day. I am going to have a great dialysis session." While this may seem a little corny or simplistic, the use of positive thinking is powerful. Once you make it a habit, it can change your life.

Another great way to keep your mind strong is to meditate on a daily basis. Ideally, you should do this several times a day, even if it's only for five minutes at a time. Turn off the radio, television, computer, cell phone, and other electronic devices, and find a quiet place. Then take a few minutes to clear your mind and reflect. In the morning, when you wake up, a brief period of meditation can bring a fresh new perspective to your day. In the middle of your day, meditation can provide a welcome break from your hectic pace, recharging you both mentally and physically. It's also a good idea to clear your mind before sleep. If you try to sleep while you're still worrying over the problems of the day, you may find your mind racing instead of "turning off." Meditation can help you relax your mind and body so that you can get some much-needed sleep.

If you have never meditated before, there are several ways in which you can go about it. The Internet offers many techniques for meditation. Just type "how to meditate" into your favorite search engine and see what comes up. You'll probably find a number of options, one of which may appeal to you. Most likely, your local library and bookstore offer a number of how-to books on the subject. You may even be able to attend a class at your local YMCA, library, adult education program, or church.

Some people find that they don't need formal step-by-step instructions to meditate. Instead, they practice simple visualization. Try sitting in a quiet room and mentally travelling to your favorite place, whether it is a deserted beach, a cool green forest, or a beautiful garden. Focus on the image while also feeling the gentle breeze and hearing the seagulls or the whisper of the trees. This, alone, can help to still your mind and easy your tension.

Another way to reach a more relaxed meditative state is to use deep breathing. I'm not talking about the unconscious "breathing reflex" that occurs all the time. I'm referring to the conscious act of breathing deeply and rhythmically. This type of breathing is vital to proper exercise and meditation, and is a form of meditation in and of itself. How do you do it? Just follow these steps.

1. Sit in a relaxed position on a chair or in bed. Using your diaphragm, breathe in deeply through your mouth for a count of five. Then hold your breath for a count of five.

2. Exhale slowly through your mouth for a count of five.

3. Repeat two or three times, each time inhaling to a count of five, holding to a count of five, and exhaling to a count of five.

After repeating this exercise several times, you will feel the tension literally dissolve from your body. I have done this exercise with patients who have come into my office with very high blood pressure, and after several minutes of slow, deep breathing, their blood pressure was significantly lower. Perhaps you remember the Chapter 6 discussion of people who begin each dialysis session with high blood pressure. (See page 85.) Using this type of meditative breathing at the beginning of each session may help you lower your blood pressure—without the use of drugs.

You may be surprised to learn that meditation doesn't have to be practiced in a sitting position. Tai Chi is perhaps the best-known form of active meditation designed for relaxation, balance, and health. Taking a daily walk can also be active meditation, as can rowing, swimming, and aquatherapy. You'll learn more about the benefits of exercise in the section that follows.

GETTING YOUR BODY IN THE GAME

Here, we are talking about the dreaded "E" word: Exercise. You now may be wondering, "Why do I need to exercise?" As you'll soon learn, the potential benefits can be great.

The Benefits of Exercise

Exercise can improve muscle strength and endurance, which is very important for some people on dialysis. It can also improve endothelial function, which, as you know from Chapter 8 (see page 114), is a major issue for most people who deal with kidney disease and dialysis. It is also a natural detoxifier. Your skin is an organ of elimination, and exercise can help you eliminate more toxins through your skin. Exercise can also improve your overall sense of well-being, and can even help you overcome an addiction such as smoking. Finally, physical activity can help get rid of "pent-up" frustration. On most forms of dialysis, you spend a significant amount of time sitting in one place. Getting up and doing something active can be just what the doctor ordered to release stress and help the body function better. Here are some other ways in which you can benefit from exercise. It can:

- Increase your energy level.

- Increase flexibility, strength, and endurance.

- Prevent the loss of muscle.

- Increase your ability to function in day-to-day activities.

- Improve your quality of sleep.

- Improve your digestion.

- Lower your cholesterol.

- Decrease the risk of heart disease.

- Lower your blood pressure.

- Reduce your blood sugar levels.

- Fight depression and enhance your sense of well-being.

The Benefits of a Physical Therapy Evaluation

When I talk to patients concerning exercise, many say, "I have difficulty walking and I have bad arthritis. I haven't exercised in years." Certainly, many people on dialysis are older and have significant health conditions, including diabetes, vascular disease, and arthritis, any of which can be debilitating. Many have difficulty walking. But in the vast majority of cases, some type of exercise is possible.

How should you start? If you haven't exercised in years, the last thing you want to do is go to a gym and put your health in the hands of a kid who is employed as a "physical fitness trainer" but doesn't understand a thing about your health problems. Instead, I strongly recommend that you get an evaluation from a physical therapist or exercise physiologist

Protecting Your Dialysis Access During Exercise

Exercise can provide you with a wealth of benefits, from improved energy to greater cardiovascular health. Be aware, though, that some types of exercise require you to safeguard your dialysis access in special ways—especially if you have an HD or PD catheter. Your access is your lifeline, so in addition to the general-care guidelines provided in Chapter 3 (see page 44), you'll want to thoroughly understand the following:

- If you have a catheter for peritoneal dialysis, you will have to clamp it off before any water exercise. Ask your healthcare team to show you how to accomplish this.

- If you have a catheter for hemodialysis, swimming is probably a no-no unless you order a special plastic cover that will maintain a tight seal around your catheter so that no water leaks in. Again, speak to your healthcare team. They will tell you what you need to get.

- Choose a chlorinated pool or ocean for your water exercise. A pond, lake, or river provides a higher risk of bacterial infection.

- As soon as you get out of the water, change the dressing on your access. You don't want it to remain wet.

- Ask your healthcare team if weightlifting is okay for you or if it will pose a danger to your access. People who have a fistula or graft usually have to avoid strenuous arm exercises. Small weights and a higher number of reps can often give you the muscle- and bone-building workout you need without damaging your access.

who has expertise in exercise and rehabilitation. Certain muscle groups— particularly those in the lower and mid-back and the abdominals—atrophy (waste away) when they haven't been used for a long period of time. The goal is to focus on those areas that need to be strengthened before you even start an exercise program. Once the muscles have been built up, your therapist can create an exercise program that is tailored to your specific needs and that can be continued at home.

How to Exercise

You've now read about the many benefits of exercise and the importance of having an evaluation if you haven't been physically active in recent years. In this section, we'll talk about the best types of exercise you can do.

Basically, a good exercise program includes two types of activity: aerobic exercise and resistance exercise. Any sustained, rhythmic exercise that is continued for a period of time is usually classified as being *aerobic*. Literally meaning "with oxygen," it increases oxygen consumption and improves cardiovascular and respiratory function, making it

Does Exercise Mean Dietary Changes?

Everyone on dialysis is aware of their dietary needs and limitations. Do these requirements and restrictions change at all when you start an exercise program? The answer is . . . maybe.

- If you exercise hard and long enough to build up a sweat, you may be able to increase your fluid intake on your exercise days. Don't do this on your own, though; discuss it with your dietitian. She may ask you to keep a log of your fluid intake and weight changes.

- You can't build muscles without protein, so if you're working out, you may need to increase your protein intake. This, too, should be talked over with your dietitian.

- Don't think that because you exercise, you can have as much sodium, potassium, and phosphorus as you like. It's still vital to follow prescribed dietary restrictions. But, of course, your monthly blood work will let your dietitian know if your diet should be "tuned up."

important for your health. This category includes swimming, aquatherapy, walking, and biking. If you have joint problems such as arthritis, swimming and aquatherapy can be especially good because they diminish the pressure on joints in the back, hips, and legs. Just be aware that water exercise makes it necessary to take special steps to protect your access. (See the inset on page 141.) Walking, too, is a wonderful choice because you can do it anywhere and move at your own pace. Biking is another great activity. Because it is non-weight-bearing, you can work out while avoiding wear and tear on your joints.

Resistance-based exercises—which include weightlifting and resistance training—work to strengthen and build muscles and increase bone strength. As you know, this is vital for people on dialysis because they tend to lose both muscle and bone mass over time.

In weightlifting, the use of low pounds and high reps is important. Your goal is not to develop huge, bulging muscles, but to become stronger and increase your muscle endurance and flexibility. When using weights, you have to be careful of your dialysis access (see the inset on page 141), and you may need to adjust your protein intake accordingly (see the inset on page 142).

The key to exercise success is choosing something you like and incorporating some degree of endurance (aerobic) and resistance-based activities. You should be as consistent as possible and try to exercise at least three times a week to start, if you are able. Begin slowly so that you don't hurt or exhaust yourself—fifteen or twenty minutes at a time is good—and build up over time. Rome wasn't built in a day, and neither are muscles or greater cardiovascular health. Any exercise you can fit into your routine is sure to improve both your physical and emotional well-being.

KEEPING YOUR SPIRIT IN THE GAME

Earlier in the chapter, we discussed steps you can take to strengthen your resolve and take charge of your life. An acceptance of your condition and a belief in your own power to make positive changes is certainly important, but it's also essential to build and fortify your spirituality—your sense of meaning, purpose, and connectedness to other people and to the universe. This connection can make an important difference by providing comfort and support whenever life throws you a "curve ball."

The Power of Prayer

Prayer is powerful. Studies have shown that people who pray experience less depression and have improved coping skills. While prayer can be a form of meditation, it is much more than that. By recognizing a higher power, you strengthen your sense of connection with the world around you and ease the burden you feel when you're dealing with a chronic illness.

If you already practice prayer, you are most likely reaping the benefits of this healing practice. If you used to pray but have not tried it in a long time, re-introduce it into your daily life. If you have never explored prayer, now is a good time to develop a spiritual life. Certainly, you can use prayers from a specific religion or creed, but you don't have to. Just find a quiet, tranquil place where you can be by yourself, and sit in a comfortable position. Try lighting a candle or playing soft music—anything that puts you at ease. Then speak to God as simply as possible. Share with him your hopes, dreams, and fears, and ask him for help and support. Although this may seem forced at first, over time, you will feel more comfortable in communicating your thoughts and feelings, and you will discover that these periods of prayer provide a feeling of serenity, an easing of burdens, and a reassuring sense of connectedness.

The Importance of Family Support

There's no doubt about it: Dialysis patients who have the support of family and friends do better. They are more likely to follow doctors' orders, they have a better quality of life, and they live longer, too. Of course, family and friends can provide practical help—rides to in-center dialysis sessions, assistance with home dialysis, and aid in preparing dialysis-friendly meals, for instance. But they offer more than that. A strong social network provides a sense of connection to the world around you—the knowledge that you are not alone. This, in turn, strengthens you both spiritually and emotionally.

Norman Cousins and the Power of Laughter

Several sections of this chapter explore the connection between mind, spirit, and body. One of the first people to make the general public aware of this link was writer Norman Cousins. While serving as editor-in-chief of the *Saturday Review* in the mid-1960s, Cousins was diagnosed with the chronic inflammatory disease ankylosing spondylitis. In severe pain, he took an unconventional approach to healing that incorporated nutritional supplementation and big doses of laughter. Cousins actually checked into a hotel room along with a supply of comedy films, including several Marx Brothers movies, and started watching one movie after another. Soon, he was laughing—and feeling much better. The laughter stimulated chemicals that not only lessened his pain but also, according to objective tests, reduced inflammation. Eventually, the editor returned to his job at the *Saturday Review* and—along with his best-selling book, *Anatomy of an Illness*—helped to usher in the holistic health revolution.

So laugh! Watch your favorite comedy films and TV shows. Read funny books. Tell jokes, and encourage the people around you to share funny stories. You may be able to laugh your way to greater wellness and a positive new attitude.

Unfortunately, many people on dialysis feel isolated by their time-consuming treatment routine and the many demands that dialysis has imposed on them, one being their dietary restrictions. They may believe that they are a burden to their family and be reluctant to ask for help. If this sounds familiar, it's important to recognize that your health depends on reaching out to the people around you. The following tips may help you connect (or re-connect) with family and friends.

- Talk to family members and friends about your health condition, and educate them about your dialysis, your diet, and anything else that you think is important. While this may feel awkward or difficult, communication is the foundation of a strong, satisfying network of support. The more the people around you know, the better able they will be to lend comfort and practical assistance.

- Provide updates for the people in your social network. If your doctor gives you bad news, don't keep it to yourself; let family and friends know about it so they can give you the support you need.

- Get involved in the lives of friends and family. They're there for you when you need them, so you should be there for them, too. Share their joys and sorrows, and make sure that all your conversations don't revolve around you and your health.

- If you don't have friends and family nearby, look into support groups. Ask your healthcare team how you can meet other patients, or search the Internet for online groups. There are plenty of people out there who know how you feel and can provide encouragement, advice, or just a sympathetic ear.

IN CONCLUSION

Dialysis brings dramatic changes to your life, but it doesn't have to change who you are. The first step in achieving greater wellness is to accept the need for treatment. Once you accept your situation, you can form a positive plan for making the best of it. Remember that you're not in this alone. To avoid feeling isolated, reach out to the people around you. Believe it or not, social support can actually make you *healthier*. Finally, strengthen your body through carefully chosen exercises. Physical activity can lessen the side effects of dialysis, release stress, enable you to better carry out daily activities, increase your energy level, and improve your overall well-being.

11

*U*nderstanding Transplantation

W hen you first noticed this chapter, you may have thought, "Why does a book on dialysis include a chapter on kidney transplants? Isn't the point of this book to tell me everything about *dialysis*?" For many people, dialysis is not an end unto itself but a bridge to transplantation. If you are medically able, your goal should be to get a transplant, which, in most cases, can improve your quality of life and also extend your life. Planning for transplantation often begins when the subject of dialysis is first addressed, so if you are on dialysis, there's a good chance that you're also thinking about a transplant.

This chapter starts by explaining what kidney transplantation is. It then discusses the different possible sources of donated kidneys, explores the lengthy evaluation process, and even looks at a new and exciting way in which some dialysis patients are finding compatible kidneys.

WHAT IS A KIDNEY TRANSPLANT?

A *kidney transplant* is a surgical procedure in which a healthy donor organ is transplanted into a patient with kidney disease. Usually, only one kidney is transplanted because a person can live a healthy life with a single functioning kidney. In rare situations, a patient receives two kidneys from a deceased donor.

Most of the time, the diseased kidneys are not removed because they pose no threat to the patient. When necessary—when the old kidneys are causing high blood pressure or are infected, for instance—the dysfunctional kidneys are removed during surgery. The new kidney is placed on the lower right or left side of the abdomen, where it can easily be connected to the blood vessels and the bladder.

WHERE DO TRANSPLANTED ORGANS COME FROM?

In any kidney transplant, the person who donates the kidney is called the *donor,* and the kidney patient who receives it is called the *recipient.* The majority of donors are deceased organ donors (cadavers) who have agreed in advance to contribute their organs or whose organs have been contributed by a parent or a spouse. Organs can also come from living donors. Basically, there are three types of donations:

- With a *cadaveric donation,* the kidney comes from a person who has passed away but has a healthy kidney that is a good match for the recipient.

- With a *living related donation,* the kidney comes from a family member—a blood relative—who is a good match for the recipient.

- With a *living unrelated donation,* the kidney comes from a close friend or, sometimes, a complete stranger who is a good match for the recipient.

As you've just learned, whether the donor is living or dead, the donated kidney has to be compatible with the person who is receiving the organ. Matching, which helps insure that the recipient's body will not reject the donor's kidney, is a complex system that can be divided into three distinct areas:

- *Blood type matching* is as important in kidney transplantation as it is in blood transfusion. There are four major human blood types—A, B, AB, and O. A type A recipient may receive a kidney from a donor with type A or O; a type B recipient may receive a kidney from a donor with type B or O; a type O recipient may receive a kidney only from a donor with blood type O; and an AB recipient can receive a kidney from a person of any blood type. The Rh factor, which adds a plus or minus before the letter, is not taken into account in kidney matching.

The Members of Your Transplant Team

In Chapter 2, you learned about the various members of the dialysis team. If you have a kidney transplant, you will have another team—one specially created to coordinate, manage, and perform your kidney transplant, and to continue care after surgery. Keep in mind that the list below includes the key players only. Transplantation is a long, complex process that begins way before the actual operation and ends long afterwards. Along the way, many doctors, nurses, and other health professionals will contribute to your care.

The Surgeon. A specially trained surgeon will determine if you are a good candidate for a kidney transplant, perform your transplant surgery, and supervise your care immediately following the operation. He may also see you in follow-up visits after your discharge from the hospital.

The Nephrologist. After surgery, you will work with a special kidney transplant doctor, who may or may not be the same nephrologist who cared for you during dialysis. You see, in the months following surgery, special medications will have to be introduced—immunosuppressants, which prevent the body's immune system from rejecting the new organ; and antibiotics and anti-fungal medications, which prevent any infection that may result from the suppression of your immune system. The nephrologist supervises the introduction and adjustment of these drugs. After six months, when your drug regimen has been established, you will probably be able to return to the care of your usual nephrologist.

The Transplant Coordinator. Usually a nurse, the transplant coordinator will work with you from your initial evaluation through in-hospital preparation, surgery, and follow-up care. He will also facilitate communication between the various members of your transplant team and any other health professionals who provide care. Usually, the coordinator is available twenty-four hours a day, seven days a week, and will be your chief support throughout the process.

The Case Manager. A case manager is a nurse or social worker who plans and monitors a transplant patient's care. Among other things, he will help you navigate the health insurance system, work with the other members of your transplant team to formulate a discharge plan that includes rehabilitation and physical therapy, and make sure that you get the medications you need after surgery.

- *Tissue matching* has to do with proteins called *antigens,* which can be identified through blood tests. Transplant professionals currently consider at least six specific antigens in each recipient and donor. The best compatibility is a six-antigen match, which occurs most frequently between siblings.

- *Crossmatching,* which can involve between ten and fifteen different tests, enables transplant professionals to better predict how a kidney recipient will respond to cells from the kidney donor. A "positive" crossmatch means that the recipient will respond to the donor by rejecting the kidney. A "negative" crossmatch is actually good; it means that the recipient will not reject the donor. Therefore, the transplant can be performed safely.

The tests that are now used to match recipients with donors are better than ever before and help contribute to the general success of kidney transplantation.

HOW ARE YOU EVALUATED FOR A KIDNEY TRANSPLANT?

Your evaluation for a kidney transplant can begin even before you have your first dialysis treatment. If you are in Stage 4 of chronic kidney disease and your glomerular filtration rate (GFR) is less than 20 mL/min (see page 8 to learn about stages), you are eligible for evaluation. The process begins with choosing a dedicated transplant center.

Finding a Dedicated Transplant Center

Although some hospitals have their own transplant centers, in most cases, you will have to go beyond your local hospital to find a dedicated facility that can perform kidney transplant evaluation and surgery. In the United States alone, there are approximately 270 dedicated transplant centers.

Your nephrologist will mostly likely recommend several facilities. Just as I have advised you to be your own healthcare advocate throughout the dialysis process, I urge you to look carefully at the available centers for kidney transplant. You can begin your search by visiting the website of Kidney Link (see page 179 of Resources) to find the centers closest to you. For each of these facilities, some of the issues you should consider include:

- How far do you have to travel to get to the transplant center? You may be willing to travel anywhere to receive topnotch care, but depending on your health and finances, travel may be a problem for you.

- How many surgeries has that particular transplant center (and that particular surgeon) performed? You want to be assured that both the center and your surgeon are highly experienced with a long record of successful transplants.

- Does that transplant center accept your insurance? This is an expensive surgery, so for most people, insurance coverage is an important issue. It's possible that the facility that's closest to you geographically does not accept your insurance.

Undergoing the Evaluation Process

Once you have selected a kidney transplant center, the evaluation can begin. Because the team at the center needs to completely understand your medical status, you will be asked a series of questions and undergo a series of tests to establish whether you're a good candidate for transplant. For instance, if you have diabetes, tests will be done to determine if your glucose levels are controlled. Other tests may include the following:

- Psychological and social evaluation.

- Blood chemistries to determine serum creatinine, electrolytes such as sodium and potassium, cholesterol, and liver function.

- Clotting studies to measure the time it takes for your blood to clot.

- Viral studies to determine if you have viruses that could increase the probability that your body will reject the donor organ. This may even include a dental evaluation to uncover infection and inflammation in the gums.

- Evaluations of cardiac function to make sure that your heart can stand up to the stresses of the surgery. At the minimum, you will have an EKG (electrocardiogram) to check the electrical activity of your heart. If there is a history of heart disease, you will probably undergo a stress test and/or cardiac catheterization.

- A lung evaluation, including a chest x-ray. If there is a history of lung disease, such as emphysema, you may be asked to see a pulmonologist for more extensive testing.

- Age-related cancer screening. For instance, if you are fifty years of age or older, you may have a colonoscopy to check your colon health. If you are male, you will have your prostate evaluated. These tests are performed because the immune system-suppressing drugs that are given to transplant patients to prevent rejection of the new kidney carry a small risk of increasing the likelihood of cancer.

- Screening for peripheral vascular disease (PVD), a blood vessel disorder that leads to narrowing and hardening of the arteries that supply the legs and feet. For a transplant to occur, the blood flow to the lower abdomen and legs needs to be adequate.

Are there factors that may prevent you from being a transplant candidate? The contraindications vary from one dialysis center to another, and may include the following:

- Active cigarette use. (Tobacco use can decrease the health of the blood vessels and increase the risk of transplant rejection.)

- Active infection.

- Active substance abuse, including alcohol and drugs.

- Active, uncontrolled psychosis.

- Advanced cirrhosis of the liver or liver failure.

- Age. (Some centers do not accept candidates who are over a certain age.)

- Body mass index (BMI) greater than 39 (very obese).

- Coronary artery disease with active cigarette use.

- Diabetes with active cigarette use.

- Heart disease that is not correctable and/or a recent heart attack.

- Lack of health insurance.

- Noncompliance with dialysis appointments and medication use.

- Recent cancer, except for non-melanotic skin cancer.

- Severe chronic obstructive pulmonary disease (COPD).

- Uncontrolled diabetes mellitus.

Getting on the Waiting List

If you are considered a kidney transplant candidate, once your specific criteria for a "match" have been determined (see page 148), you will be placed on a waiting list for a compatible kidney. In the United States, the United Network for Organ Sharing (UNOS) oversees the allocation of not only kidneys, but all types of organs, including liver, pancreas, heart, lung, and cornea. UNOS receives information from hospitals and medical centers throughout the country regarding adults and children who need transplants. Your medical transplant team is responsible for sending your data to UNOS and keeping it updated if and when your medical status changes. Those individuals who are in most urgent need of transplant are placed highest on the list and given priority. (To learn more about UNOS, visit their website, which is provided on page 180 of the Resources list.)

When a donor kidney becomes available, the UNOS computer searches the people on the waiting list for a recipient who is a good match. Although people with a high priority are considered first, sometimes, people lower on the list receive the available kidney because of factors such as the size of the donor organ and the geographic distance between the donor and the kidney recipient.

As more people are diagnosed with advanced kidney disease, more people are added to the UNOS waiting list. In 2011, more than 16,000 kidney-alone transplants were performed in the United States, but as of this writing, over 90,000 people are waiting to receive a kidney. The average wait is two to three years. That's why it's so important to get on the UNOS list as soon as possible.

Kidney Exchanges—A New Way to Cut the Waiting Time

A friend or family member who is willing to make a donation of a kidney can literally save the life of someone with advanced kidney disease. The problem has long been that the donated kidney is not always a match for the recipient. In 2010, though, the United Network for Organ Sharing (UNOS) began a nationally run exchange program that allows "kidney paired donations." Basically, a relative or friend makes a kidney donation on the patient's behalf, and the patient, in return, receives a compatible kidney from another living donor.

Before 2010, some transplant centers were able to mix and match large numbers of patients and donors. The nationwide UNOS database promises to make these matches more widely available, with some experts predicting that it could result in an additional 2,000 to 3,000 transplants a year. By increasing the donor pool and removing some people from the national waiting list, this is good news even for patients who do not have living donors.

As you learned earlier in the chapter, the people closest to you—family and friends—can donate a kidney, enabling you to get a transplant without going through a potentially long waiting period. When these donors are not a good match—which happens about a third of the time—a new national database can often arrange a "swap" that, in effect, trades the donor kidney for one that's more compatible. (See the inset at the top of this page.)

IS KIDNEY TRANSPLANTATION A "CURE"?

A kidney transplant replaces your dysfunctional kidneys with a functioning organ, making it unnecessary to have your blood artificially filtered through dialysis. However, a transplant should not be regarded as a "cure," but as a treatment option—albeit, usually the *best* treatment option currently available. The great majority of people enjoy better quality of life after getting a new kidney. Just be aware that once you have a transplant, you will have to be diligent in taking your immunosuppressive medication for the rest of your life, and you will have to see a kidney doctor on a regular basis.

IN CONCLUSION

This chapter provided only a brief overview of the kidney transplant process. From the time you begin evaluation to the time you actually receive your new kidney, years may elapse. Because this process can take a long time, you should begin your evaluation as soon as you are eligible. For those who are eligible, the kidney transplant is the gold standard of treatment.

12

Ten Ways to Improve Your Dialysis Sessions

The first eleven chapters of this book were designed to increase your understanding of kidney disease and kidney dialysis, and let you know about the many ways in which you can improve your health and well-being throughout your treatments. By now, your head may be swimming with all the different aspects of self-care. Certainly, I encourage you to learn everything you can and (eventually) take all the steps, big and small, that will strengthen your body, mind, and spirit. But you may be wondering if certain steps will have an *especially* significant impact on your health. Absolutely! This chapter homes in on ten major ways in which you can improve your dialysis sessions, your daily life, and your overall health.

1. Choose a Home-Based Dialysis Option

In general, people do better on home-based modalities. Home dialysis will give you a greater sense of control over your health and everyday life. You won't have to travel back and forth to a dialysis center, and you will be able to arrange your treatment sessions around your activities rather than re-arranging your life to accommodate your medical facility's schedule. When you can dialyze at home, you can also dialyze more often, which means that your fluids will be better managed, you'll have fewer dietary restrictions, and you'll probably enjoy a better overall sense of well-being. (To learn more about the different modes of home-based dialysis, turn to page 22 of Chapter 2.)

Perhaps in the past, you heard stories about home dialysis being difficult. If that's what's keeping you from exploring this option, be aware that the current dialysis machines are easier to set up and use than the older ones. Also, you'll be allowed to manage your own care only when you're considered ready to do so, so there's no need to fear that you won't be able to handle it. You will get sufficient training and will also receive ongoing support from a dialysis nurse.

Is home dialysis for everyone? No. But if it's possible in your case, try to be open to this great alternative.

2. If You Opt for In-Center Dialysis, Choose Nocturnal Treatments

If home-based treatments are not a good option for you, consider nocturnal dialysis. I know several patients who felt worn-out on standard hemodialysis and did far better after switching to nocturnal sessions. Because these longer treatments remove more toxins and fluids—and eliminate them more gently over a longer period of time—people feel healthier and more energetic, need less medication, and have fewer dietary restrictions. Nocturnal treatments are especially good for patients who are larger or who tend to gain a lot of fluids between treatments.

Is nocturnal dialysis second on my list because it's not as good as home-based therapy? Absolutely not. Nocturnal treatments provide an excellent level of care. The issue is simply that you have to spend three nights a week at a dedicated dialysis center. For some people, this is too much time spent away from home. (To learn more about this mode of dialysis, turn to page 23.)

Before we leave the topic of dialysis treatment options, let me be perfectly clear: I am *not* against three-times-a-week in-center dialysis. There are many people who use it and feel great. If it works for you, I'm truly glad that you are doing so well. For some people, though, these short sessions, in which large amounts of fluids are removed fairly quickly, lead to unpleasant drops in blood pressure, exhaustion, and a variety of disagreeable symptoms. It's good to know that there are other options available.

Examine Your Options

At the dialysis unit where I do rounds, on three days each week, the unit is open for twenty-four hours. On those days, in addition to the regular morning and afternoon shifts, there is an evening session that accommodates people with daytime jobs. The center also tries to be flexible for those patients who want nocturnal HD; they can start early and still have a six- to eight-hour treatment. We offer these options so that each patient can work around her activities and have greater control over her life.

If you currently have daytime dialysis sessions but find that they are interfering with your job or your social activities—or if you think that you might feel better if you had longer sessions—talk to your dialysis center about the possibility of evening treatments. If your current center doesn't offer this type of flexibility, see if there are other nearby centers that can be more accommodating. Changing your treatment hours can make a big difference to both your health and the quality of your day-to-day life.

3. Know and Understand Your Dry Weight

As you learned in Chapter 6, your *estimated dry weight (EDW)* is your weight without excess fluid. (See page 79 for more information.) Your EDW is important, because it is the difference between this weight and your weight as measured before a dialysis session that determines how the dialysis machine is set. The greater the difference between the two numbers, the more fluid will be removed by the machine during your treatment.

Why am I explaining this? If, during dialysis, you experience cramping and signs of low blood pressure such as dizziness and nausea, and if after each session, you feel tired and lethargic, it may be because a large volume of fluid is being filtered out during a very short period of time. This can mean that that you're gaining too much fluid between treatments (turn to page 160 to learn more about that), or it may mean that your estimated dry weight is too low. To put it another way, it's possible that the machine is being set to remove more fluids than is actually necessary or healthy. As the word "estimated" implies, there's no way to precisely determine dry weight. But if you're diligent about minimizing fluid gain between treatments and you still suffer disabling side effects during dialysis, you should speak to your doctor about raising your dry weight. This one change may make a tremendous difference in the way you feel.

4. Minimize Your Fluid Gains

Above, I discussed the unpleasant side effects you may experience when a large amount of fluid is removed during a standard dialysis session. As explained, this sometimes occurs because the estimated dry weight is too low, but it can also occur because excessive fluids have been gained between treatments. And excessive fluid gain can do far more damage than making your dialysis experience unpleasant. It can cause high blood pressure, edema (swelling), shortness of breath, and even serious heart problems such as congestive heart failure. That's why it's so important to minimize fluid gains.

Many people are able to reduce fluid gains by limiting sodium intake and restricting fluids. (See page 81 of Chapter 6 for more information.) If you have residual kidney function—in other words, if you still produce some urine—the use of diuretics may also be helpful. (See page 97 of Chapter 7.) Some people, though, find it very difficult to control fluid gain as long as they remain on standard three-times-a-week hemodialysis. If you are among these people, nocturnal HD or a home dialysis option—peritoneal dialysis or home HD—may be just what you need.

5. Remember That Nutrition Matters

Your diet is of paramount importance. As you learned in Chapter 9, people on dialysis need a good supply of high-quality proteins such as lean meat and poultry, fish, and egg whites. Both your weight and your albumin level, which is tested in your monthly blood work, are good indications of whether you are getting all the protein you need. If, over a three- to four-week period, you find that you are losing weight or that your albumin is down, you should have a serious discussion with your renal dietitian. Perhaps you can change your diet to include more protein, or perhaps you need a protein supplement. (See page 116 of Chapter 8 to learn more about this.)

Low albumin can indicate not just low protein but also inflammation, so if your albumin level continues to be a problem, you should discuss the possibility of infection with your nephrologist. You can eat all the protein that you want, but if an infection is present, your body may not be able to utilize the protein properly. The problem of inflammation is another reason to carefully choose your foods. A good dialysis diet supplies not just protein, but also healthy amounts of inflammation-fighting fruits and vegetables. Just make sure that the fruits and veggies you choose are low in potassium. (See page 127 for lists of low- and high-potassium foods.)

Finally, you must work with your dietitian to create a plan that meets all of your nutritional needs and avoids or limits substances that your body may not be able to handle. Chapter 9 provides a good deal of information on an appropriate dialysis diet, but nothing can replace the specific guidance that your renal dietitian prepares based on your medical condition and your monthly blood work.

6. Take Supplements That Enhance Energy and Overall Health

Throughout this book, I've mentioned that one of the biggest complaints of people on dialysis is fatigue. Sometimes a patient's exhaustion is so debilitating that she ends up quitting her job, abandoning her hobbies, and skipping get-togethers with family and friends. Needless to say, this ailment can have an enormous impact on quality of life.

The loss of energy experienced by dialysis patients can have a number of causes, including anemia, uremia, the effects of dialysis, and poor nutrition. Although all of these issues should be addressed, I've found that many patients can greatly benefit from nutritional supplements that enable the body to produce more energy. In Chapter 8, you learned about a number of these supplements. (See page 102.) But when a patient complains about fatigue and is unwilling to add more than a few pills to her daily medication regimen, I usually prescribe the three most important energy-enhancing supplements: coenzyme Q_{10} (CoQ_{10}), L-carnitine, and D-ribose.

In most cases, I recommend starting with 100 mg of CoQ_{10} taken twice a day, 500 mg of L-carnitine taken every other day, and 2,000 mg of D-ribose taken every other day. I then gradually increase the level of L-carnitine to 1,000 mg every day. If you've read Chapter 8, you may remember that these supplements offer benefits beyond greater energy. They can also help lower blood pressure and blood glucose levels.

Although my experience has shown that these supplements can make a vast improvement in people's lives, I must remind you that no supplements should be added to your regimen without the okay of your nephrologist, who can best determine if these nutrients are right for you.

7. Use a Kidney-Based Probiotic

Throughout this book, I have explained that even if you use home hemodialysis or daily peritoneal dialysis, your treatments cannot filter out waste products as well as functioning kidneys would. Yes, they remove many of the uremic toxins that accumulate in the body, but they cannot remove all of them. This is one of the reasons that a probiotic specially designed for people with kidney problems can be so beneficial. This supplement, which contains "good" bacteria, can break down many of the remaining toxic substances and metabolize them so that the body can eliminate them through the bowel. This, in turn, reduces the body's inflammatory response, resulting in a healthier body and a greater sense of overall well-being.

In addition to helping to break down and eliminate toxins, a kidney-specific probiotic also offers the benefits most often associated with this class of supplements: It helps normalize bowel flora (microorganisms) and bowel function, and prevents the overgrowth of *Candida albicans*, a microorganism that can cause infection.

Probiotics are usually well tolerated by people on dialysis. I generally recommend starting with one capsule per meal per day, and after a couple of weeks, increasing the dose to two capsules per meal. (For more information on probiotics, see page 108 of Chapter 8.)

8. Take Steps to Correct Your Acidosis

As you learned in Chapter 1 (see page 7), healthy kidneys help maintain the body's acid/alkaline balance through use of an alkalizing substance known as bicarbonate. When the kidneys no longer function and are unable to perform their "balancing act," the body becomes too acidic. This weakens all the body systems, including the immune system, and promotes inflammation. Dialysis does help control acidosis, but again, it cannot do the work of healthy kidneys.

A great way to restore acid-alkaline balance is to drink water that has been processed through a system that filters out contaminants, adds important minerals, and makes the water slightly alkaline. (See page 179 of the Resources section.) You can also enjoy homemade alkalizing juices, such as a combination of kale, carrots, and apples. Finally, be sure to make alkalizing fruits and vegetables part of your diet. Good choices include berries, broccoli, cherries, lettuce, onions, bell peppers, and pineapple. Of course, you'll want to avoid or greatly limit fruits and veggies that are high in potassium. By taking steps to correct your body's acidosis, you will do a great deal to promote your overall health.

9. Take Care of Your Dialysis Access

As you learned in Chapter 3, your dialysis access—whether a fistula, a graft, or a catheter—is your lifeline. It is vital that you learn how to care for your access, not only on dialysis days, but also on non-dialysis days. Learn to check for the *thrill*—a vibration or pulse which shows that blood is flowing unimpeded through the access. Keep the area clean and protect it from water. Be alert to signs of infection and other common problems. Protect your access arm by not using it to carry heavy items, by not sleeping on it, and by wearing loose-fitting clothing. (For detailed instructions on access care, turn to page 44 in Chapter 3.)

You can also help maintain your access by taking nutritional supplements that can enhance the health of your blood vessels, including the blood vessels that were used to create your fistula or graft. A good supplement regimen that includes at least 50 mg of resveratrol (see page 114), and perhaps 200 to 400 mg of turmeric (page 106) and 500 mg of quercetin (page 107), can do a great deal to keep both your blood vessels and your access in good condition. Just be sure to okay these supplements with your nephrologist.

10. Avoid Boredom During Dialysis Sessions

Most people on dialysis spend hours at a time confined to a chair or bed during treatments. While this can be tedious or even depressing, it does not have to be. There is a lot you can do to keep yourself interested and entertained—and, perhaps, even productive—during dialysis. The following list is sure to provide a few appealing ideas. Just keep in mind that although technological advances provide more entertainment and communication options than ever before, many dialysis units do not allow you to plug your own devices into their electrical outlets. There is a good reason for this: The center wants to make sure that your devices do not interrupt the flow of electricity to the unit's lifesaving equipment or in any way interfere with its proper function. Check your unit's policy, and if there are rules against "plugging in," make sure that your devices are fully charged and that you always have some backup activities that don't require electricity or batteries.

- **Watch TV.** Most, although not all, units provide a television for every patient. While this may not keep you amused for the entire dialysis session, it will certainly provide a lot of entertainment options.

- **Read a book.** If you love reading, books can make your dialysis sessions far more pleasant and even educational. You can, of course, take along a traditional "paper" book, or you can choose an e-reader such as a Kindle, Nook, or iPad. These options are light, easy to carry, and in many cases, will permit you to choose a new book within moments of finishing the old one. (They may also give you access to newspapers and magazines.) Be aware that while there are plenty of devices designed especially for reading, free software can turn just about any laptop computer, tablet, or smart phone into an e-reader. If the cost of the individual books is an issue, check with your local library about electronic books that can be downloaded free of charge.

- **Listen to a book.** Some people find it easier or more pleasurable to listen to a book rather than reading one. Libraries offer books on CD and cassette, giving you plenty of choices. Some e-readers also have "read aloud" functions that turn e-books into spoken books. Headphones will keep your book from bothering your "neighbors."

- **Listen to music.** Depending on your selection, music can entertain, energize, or promote relaxation. Some of the devices that can provide your favorite sounds include cassette players, CD players, MP3 players, and iPods. Again, you'll want to use headphones.

- **Watch a movie.** Some dialysis centers have TVs that are connected to the Internet. This can enable you to watch the movie of your choice without toting around your own electronics. If your unit doesn't provide this, take along a fully charged laptop, tablet, smart phone, or portable DVD player.

- **Play a game.** If you love games, there are many ways in which you can enjoy them during your sessions. You can, of course, bring along tried-and-true "paper" puzzles, such as crossword and Sudoku, but technology offers many more alternatives. If you have a smart phone or just about any other electronic device, you'll find an almost endless list of game applications and websites, many of which are free.

- **Knit, crochet, needlepoint, or embroider.** While it can be a challenge to work on handicrafts with one arm connected to a dialysis machine, many patients manage to produce beautiful items while keeping themselves occupied. Smaller projects, like scarves, are easier to control around all that tubing.

- **Keep in touch with family and friends.** Whether you want to pen an old-fashioned letter or communicate via email, you'll have plenty of time to connect with relatives and friends during your treatment sessions. If you join Facebook, you might even make some new friends.

- **Learn.** Through books, CD players, iPods, and an ever-increasing number of electronic devices, you can learn a new language, explore a new hobby, or even take a college course. The possibilities are endless.

IN CONCLUSION

This chapter has focused on a number of important ways in which you can make your dialysis treatments more comfortable, enhance your health through diet and nutritional supplements, help build mental and spiritual soundness, and increase your enjoyment of daily life. By taking an active role in your own care and being aware of the many steps that can improve your health and happiness, you can truly thrive on dialysis.

Conclusion

This book provides a wealth of information on dialysis, including why and when it is used, how it works, how it can be provided, and how it may affect you. Most important, it offers the facts, guidance, and insights you need to make the best possible choices regarding every aspect of your care, from dialysis and medication to diet and nutritional supplements. As you've learned, a number of decisions lay ahead of you. What type of dialysis will you use? Will you have your treatments at home or at a dedicated dialysis center, during the day or at night? What other steps will you take to improve your physical condition and your mental and spiritual well-being? While some of these issues may seem intimidating, I urge you to view each one, large and small, as an opportunity to change things for the better.

When you learned that you needed dialysis, you might have felt helpless, but the truth is that you are far from helpless. Whether you are just considering dialysis or have already begun treatment, there is, in fact, an arsenal of health-promoting weapons at your disposal. In this book, I have tried to make you aware of them.

Of course, learning about your options is just the first step. Now, you must take action. Start by talking to your doctor so that you can ask relevant questions about your treatment—questions that will yield the information you need about your specific condition and requirements. Work with your renal dietitian to create an eating plan that will maximize your well-being. Keep an eye on your monthly blood work so that you can evaluate the effects of your dialysis sessions, medications, and food choices. Take the best possible care of your access. Always keep your dialysis team informed of how you feel during and between treatments. And take all the steps you can to strengthen not only your body, but also your mind and spirit. Even seemingly small steps, such as beginning each dialysis session with a few minutes of deep breathing or taking a daily walk, can make a huge difference in the way you feel.

This book has put the power of change in your hands, and I urge you to be proactive in your search for greater health and a more satisfying life. Never stop learning about dialysis options, never stop learning about ways in which you can enhance your well-being, and never doubt your ability to survive and thrive on dialysis. If you have further questions or you just want to fill me in on your progress, please visit my website at www.improveyourkidneyhealth.com. I look forward to hearing from you.

$\mathcal{G}$lossary

All words that appear in *italic type* are defined within the glossary.

access. In *dialysis*, a specially created entryway into the bloodstream (for *hemodialysis*) or the abdominal cavity (for *peritoneal dialysis*) that allows the blood to be filtered. Depending on the type of dialysis chosen and the patient's physical condition, the access can take the form of a *fistula*, *graft*, *hemodialysis catheter*, or *peritoneal catheter*.

acidosis. A condition in which the body fluids become too acidic. In *chronic kidney disease* and *dialysis*, acidosis occurs because the kidneys are unable to excrete excess acids and because the body's levels of *bicarbonate* fall.

albumin. A protein made by the liver and found in the blood. Causes of low albumin levels can include an inadequate consumption of calories or protein, or the presence of *inflammation*.

anabolic state. A state in which the building up and repair of tissues predominates in the body. See also *catabolic state*.

anemia. A deficiency of *red blood cells*, which are the oxygen-carrying components of the blood. People with kidney disease often have anemia because diseased kidneys are unable to make a sufficient amount of the hormone *erythropoietin*, which stimulates the bone marrow to produce red blood cells.

aneurysm. An abnormal enlargement or ballooning of a blood vessel caused by a weakening of the vessel's walls.

antioxidants. Substances that counteract or neutralize the effects of *free radicals* (unstable molecules) and can therefore help prevent cancer, heart disease, and many other disorders. Well-known antioxidants include vitamin C, vitamin E, and beta-carotene.

aortic stenosis. A condition in which the opening of the aortic valve of the heart is narrowed, decreasing the flow of blood from the heart to the rest of the body.

arteriovenous (AV) fistula. See *fistula.*

automated peritoneal dialysis (APD). A form of *peritoneal dialysis* in which a machine called a *cycler* is programmed to automatically fill the abdomen with the *dialysate* and, after a period of time called the *dwell time,* drain it out of the abdomen.

autonomic nervous system. The portion of the nervous system that controls involuntary functions of the body, such as the narrowing or widening of blood vessels and the rate at which the heart beats. This system consists of two major complementary divisions—the *sympathetic nervous system* and the *parasympathetic nervous system.*

bicarbonate. An *electrolyte* that helps keep the pH of the blood from becoming too acidic.

blood pressure. The pressure exerted by the blood against the blood vessels as the heart pumps. A blood pressure reading is made up of two numbers. The upper number, or systolic pressure, shows the pressure at the peak of a heartbeat. The lower number, or diastolic pressure, shows the pressure between heartbeats.

bruit. In *dialysis,* a whooshing sound—heard through use of a stethoscope—indicating that blood is flowing through the *access.*

buttonhole technique. A technique in which a tunnel of scar tissue is created under the skin to make the insertion of *dialysis* needles into the *access* more easy and comfortable.

cadaveric donation. The donation of a kidney by a person who has passed away but is a good match for the recipient.

calcimimetic. A medication that mimics the action of calcium on the body. This class of drugs decreases the secretion of the *parathyroid hormone* (PTH) and is often used to treat *hyperparathyroidism.*

catabolic state. A state in which the breaking down of tissues predominates in the body. See also *anabolic state.*

catheter. See *hemodialysis catheter; peritoneal catheter.*

chronic kidney disease (CKD). A gradual loss of kidney function that is usually permanent. This disorder is defined in terms of five stages, with Stage 1 being the least severe and Stage 5 indicating kidney failure.

congestive heart failure. A condition in which the heart can't pump enough blood to meet the needs of the body. This disorder can lead to a buildup of fluid in the lungs and the surrounding tissues.

continual ambulatory peritoneal dialysis (CAPD). A form of *peritoneal dialysis* in which you manually fill the abdomen with the *dialysate,* and, after a period of time called the *dwell time,* manually drain the *dialysate* out of the abdomen.

coronary heart disease (CHD). Also called coronary artery disease, a narrowing of the blood vessels that supply blood and oxygen to the heart caused by the buildup of plaque inside the vessels. Chronic kidney disease is a risk factor for the development of CHD.

creatinine. A waste product of muscle metabolism that is measured to determine kidney function and to calculate the *glomerular filtration rate (GFR).*

cycler. In *automated peritoneal dialysis (APD),* the machine that automatically removes old *dialysate* from the abdomen and replaces it with new *dialysate.*

dialysate. A special chemical solution used in *hemodialysis* and *peritoneal dialysis* to draw toxic wastes and excess fluids out of the bloodstream. Different dialysates, with different chemical compositions, are used for different types of dialysis and/or to meet the individual needs of the patient. After treatment, the dialysate is discarded along with the toxins it removed.

dialysis. The process of filtering toxins and excess fluids from the blood, usually through the use of a machine. There are two major forms of dialysis—*hemodialysis* (HD) and *peritoneal dialysis* (PD).

dialysis access. See *access.*

diffusion. The process through which particles move through a *semipermeable membrane* from an area of higher concentration to an area of lower concentration. It is through this process that toxins are removed from the blood during *dialysis.*

diuretics. Medications that relieve the buildup of excess fluids by increasing the discharge of urine. Diuretics are often used in the treatment of high blood pressure, kidney disease, and heart disease.

dwell time. In *peritoneal dialysis (PD),* the period of time during which the dialysis solution, or *dialysate,* remains in the stomach before being drained.

edema. Excess fluid trapped in the body's tissues. Most often seen as swelling in the arms, hands, legs, ankles, and feet, edema is a common symptom of kidney disease.

electrolytes. Minerals that conduct electrical impulses in the body and are vital in the control of fluids, the generation of energy, and many other important biochemical reactions. The body's major electrolytes include *bicarbonate,* calcium, chloride, magnesium, phosphate, potassium, sodium, and sulfate.

end stage renal disease (ESRD). Stage 5 of *chronic kidney disease,* in which there is complete or almost complete failure of kidney function. This condition is also called end stage kidney disease, renal failure, and kidney failure.

endothelial cells. The cells that line the interior of the blood vessels throughout the body. These cells take part in a number of vital functions, including the control of blood pressure.

erythropoietin. A hormone produced by the kidneys that promotes the formation of *red blood cells* by the bone marrow.

erythropoietin-stimulating agents (ESAs). Medications designed to stimulate the bone marrow to make *red blood cells.*

estimated dry weight (EDW). An individual's weight without excess fluids.

exchange. In *peritoneal dialysis (PD),* the process of draining old *dialysate* from the abdomen and replacing it with new *dialysate.*

exit site. In a discussion of *catheters,* the area where the catheter and skin surface make contact.

ferritin level. A test that measures the blood level of the protein ferritin as a means of measuring the amount of iron stored in the body.

fistula. A type of *dialysis access* in which a connection is surgically made between an artery and a vein, without the use of any artificial material. Also called an arteriovenous (AV) fistula, it is considered the best overall access for *hemodialysis*.

fluid overload. A buildup of fluids in the body. Also called hypervolemia and volume overload, common symptoms include an increase in body weight, *edema*, and shortness of breath. It can occur as a result of kidney disease, *congestive heart failure*, or both. In advanced kidney disease, fluid overload can be a reason to start dialysis.

free radicals. Unstable, highly reactive molecules that are created in the body through normal physiological processes as well as exposure to toxic substances. These molecules can damage cells and are believed to play a part in the development and progression of cancer, heart disease, and many other health disorders.

glomerular filtration rate (GFR). A measure of how well the kidneys are filtering toxic waste products out of the blood. Specifically, based on the level of the waste product *creatinine,* the GFR estimates how much blood passes through the kidneys' tiny filters (the glomeruli) each minute.

graft. A type of *dialysis access* created by indirectly connecting an artery to a vein through a synthetic tube that allows the blood to flow from one vessel to the other.

hematocrit. The percentage of whole blood composed of *red blood cells.*

hemodialysis (HD). A medical procedure in which waste products and excess fluids are filtered out of the blood through use of a special dialysis machine.

hemodialysis catheter. A small, flexible tube that is inserted in a vein to permit access to the bloodstream for the purpose of *dialysis.*

hemoglobin. The protein in *red blood cells* that carries oxygen throughout the body.

home hemodialysis (home HD). *Hemodialysis* that is performed at the patient's home, usually by the patient and/or a helper. It is generally performed four to five times a week, with each session lasting for two and a half to three and a half hours.

hyperglycemia. An abnormally high level of blood sugar (glucose).

hyperparathyroidism. Excessive production of the *parathyroid hormone* (PTH). This condition can lead to a weakening of the bones due to the loss of bone calcium and phosphorus.

hypertension. A condition in which the flow of blood against artery walls is high enough to eventually cause health problems such as heart disease. This condition is also called high blood pressure.

hypoglycemia. An abnormally low level of blood sugar (glucose).

hypotension. A condition in which the flow of blood against artery walls is low enough to cause symptoms such as dizziness or fainting, or even be life-threatening. This condition is also called low blood pressure.

immunosuppressant drug. A medication that inhibits activity of the immune system. This class of medications is used after a kidney transplant to prevent the recipient's body from producing antibodies that would reject the transplanted organ.

in-center dialysis. *Hemodialysis* that is performed in a dedicated dialysis facility. Standard in-center dialysis is usually performed three times a week, with each session lasting about four hours. *Nocturnal dialysis* is usually performed three nights a week, with each session lasting from six to eight hours.

inflammation. A protective tissue response—often involving pain, heat, and swelling—that usually results from illness or trauma. Although acute inflammation is a necessary part of the recovery process, chronic inflammation is harmful to the body over time and is associated with many common illnesses, including chronic kidney disease.

iron saturation level. A test measuring how much iron is circulating in the blood. It is used to detect iron excess or deficiency.

kidney transplant. A surgical procedure in which a healthy donor organ is transplanted into a patient with kidney disease.

Kt/V. A test performed to determine how well dialysis is clearing urea from the body.

living related donation. The donation of a kidney by a family member (blood relative) who is a good match for the recipient.

living unrelated donation. The donation of a kidney by a close friend or complete stranger who is a good match for the recipient.

nephrologist. A medical doctor who specializes in the care of the kidneys and the treatment of kidney disorders.

nocturnal dialysis (ND). *Hemodialysis* that is performed in a dedicated dialysis facility on a nighttime schedule. Usually, it is done three nights a week, with each session lasting from six to eight hours.

non-dominant arm. The arm that is used least frequently (e.g., the left arm of a right-handed person). Generally, a fistula or graft is placed in the patient's non-dominant arm.

parasympathetic nervous system. The portion of the *autonomic nervous system* that acts to slow the heart rate, lower blood pressure, and otherwise return the body to a balanced state after it has experienced pain or other stress. See also *sympathetic nervous system.*

parathyroid hormone. Secreted by the cells of the parathyroid gland, a substance that controls levels of calcium, phosphorus, and vitamin D in the bones and blood.

peritoneal catheter. A small, flexible tube that is inserted through the abdominal wall and into the abdominal (peritoneal) cavity for the purpose of *dialysis.*

peritoneal dialysis (PD). A medical procedure in which waste products and excess fluid are filtered out of the blood through use of the peritoneal membrane, which is a semipermeable membrane that lines the abdominal cavity. There are two types of PD—*continual ambulatory peritoneal dialysis (CAPD)* and *automated peritoneal dialysis (APD).*

peritonitis. An *inflammation* of the peritoneum (the lining of the abdominal cavity), usually caused by bacterial infection.

phosphorus binder. Also called a phosphate binder, a medication used to reduce the body's absorption of the mineral phosphorus so that it does not build up to toxic levels.

probiotics. Live cultures of "good" bacteria that are normally found in the digestive system.

pruritis. Intense chronic itching, often associated with *uremia.*

red blood cells. The blood cells that carry *hemoglobin*, which allows them to transport oxygen throughout the body.

residual kidney function. Also called residual renal function, the remaining ability of diseased kidneys to perform some filtering of the blood. Even in the case of kidney failure, there may still be some residual kidney function.

semipermeable membrane. A membrane that allows the passage of some substances from one solution to another, but does not permit the passage of other substances. *Hemodialysis* makes use of an artificial (manmade) membrane, while *peritoneal dialysis* makes use of a natural membrane (the lining of the abdominal cavity).

stenosis. The abnormal narrowing of a passage in the body. For dialysis patients, the stenosis of a vein or artery can make it impossible to place or properly develop a dialysis *access* such as a *fistula* or *graft*.

subcutaneous injection. The injection of a fluid under the skin.

sympathetic nervous system. The portion of the *autonomic nervous system* that acts to increase heart rate, raise blood pressure, and otherwise allow the body to function under stress. See also *parasympathetic nervous system*.

thrill. In *dialysis,* a vibration or pulse—felt by placing a hand over the *access*—indicating that blood is flowing through the access.

ultrafiltration. The part of the *dialysis* process that removes excess fluid from the blood.

urea reduction ratio (URR). A test performed to determine how well dialysis is clearing urea from the body.

uremia. A toxic condition characterized by a buildup of bloodstream waste products that are normally excreted in the urine. Usually occurring in end stage (Stage 5) kidney disease or when the *glomerular filtration rate* (GFR) is less than 10 mL/min (or kidney function is less than 10 percent), symptoms can include nausea, vomiting, metallic taste, fatigue, *pruritus,* and/or hiccups. This condition often indicates a need to begin *dialysis*.

vein mapping. In *dialysis,* a special ultrasound imaging test used to determine if the veins close to the surface of the skin are suitable for the placement of a *fistula* or *graft*.

white blood cells (WBCs). Also called leukocytes, the nearly colorless cells that kill bacteria, combat disease, fight allergic reactions, and destroy old and damaged cells.

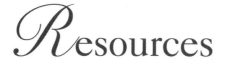

$\mathscr{R}$esources

A number of organizations and websites provide a wealth of information on kidney disease, different forms of dialysis, nutrition, medication, transplantation, and other subjects of interest to the person who is preparing for or already receiving dialysis treatments. Below, you'll find a listing of these organizations. Also included are companies that offer high-quality drinking water systems, nutritional supplements, and other dialysis-related products and services.

CHRONIC KIDNEY DISEASE, DIALYSIS, AND NUTRITION INFORMATION

American Association of Kidney Patients (AAKP)

3505 E. Frontage Road, Suite 315
Tampa, FL 33607
Phone: 800-749-2257
Website: www.aakp.org

A national nonprofit organization founded by kidney patients for kidney patients, the AAKP is dedicated to improving the lives of those who have chronic kidney disease, are undergoing dialysis, or are exploring kidney transplantation. The website provides a wealth of information on these topics.

American Kidney Fund (AKF)

11921 Rockville Pike, Suite 300
Rockville, MD 20852
Phone: 800-638-8299

Website: www.kidneyfund.org

The American Kidney Fund is a national organization that not only helps fight kidney disease through education, but also provides monetary support for those who need help in meeting the costs associated with the treatment of kidney failure. Patients requiring treatment-related financial assistance can speak to their dialysis center social worker for information about patient grants.

Davita Dialysis
1551 Wewatta Street
Denver, CO 80202
Phone: 303-405-2100
Website: www.davita.com

A leading dialysis provider, DaVita, through its extensive website, offers helpful information on kidney disease and treatment modalities, provides online discussion forums, and posts kidney-friendly recipes.

Fresenius Medical Care
920 Winter Street
Waltham, MA 02451-1457
Phone: 800-662-1237
Website: www.fmcna.com

A leading dialysis provide, Fresnius offers dialysis services and renal care products, including dialysis machines.

Improve Your Kidney Health.com
Website: www.improveyourkidneyhealth.com

Designed to provide you with up-to-date information, this website offers links to information on kidney disease, dialysis, and other topics of interest, as well the Improve Your Kidney Health Blog.

National Kidney Foundation (NKF)
30 East 33rd Street
New York, NY 10016
Phone: 800-622-9010
Website: www.kidney.org

Dedicated to enhancing the lives of people who are at risk for or are affected by kidney disease, the NKF explores many topics of interest through its website. Use the "Search" feature on the home page to find nutritional guidelines and other helpful information.

The Nephron Information Center Food Values

Website: www.foodvalues.us

This site offers nutritional information sourced from the USDA. Simply type in the name of the food or select a category, and get results. Do not overlook the links that are almost hidden in the upper right-hand corner of the website. Click on "Renal Nutrition" for a wealth of data, including an introduction to renal nutrition, and dialysis mode-specific nutritional guidelines.

Self Nutrition Data

Website: www.nutritiondata.com

This website explores a range of nutrition topics, such as diabetes and heart health. It also enables you to generate lists of foods that are high or low in a particular nutrient, and provides complete nutritional data—including potassium, sodium, and phosphorus—for individual foods, both plain and prepared. (Just plug the name of the food into the "Search" feature, and you will be able to choose from a long list of items.)

HEALTHY DRINKING WATER SYSTEMS

Santevia Water Systems

203-4841 Delta Street
British Columbia, Canada
Phone: 866-943-9200
Website: www.santevia.com

Santevia supplies alkaline water systems that clean, mineralize, and energize water, while adjusting the pH balance to mildly alkaline.

KIDNEY TRANSPLANTATION INFORMATION

Kidney Link

Website: www.kidneylink.org

Kidney Link was designed as a "kidney transplant navigator." In addition to offering information on the transplant process, types of donations, and more, the website provides a handy "Locator" service that generates a list of transplant centers in your area.

Living Kidney Donors Network

Phone: 312-473-3772
Website: www.lkdn.org

Created by Harvey Mysel, himself a kidney transplant recipient, the LKDN is a not-for-profit organization dedicated to educating people with kidney disease about the living donation process and helping them communicate with family and friends.

United Network for Organ Sharing (UNOS)
PO Box 2484
Richmond, VA 23218
Phone: 888-894-6361
Website: www.unos.org

A private, not-for-profit organization, UNOS works with the federal government to manage the nation's organ transplant system. The "Patient Education" section of its website provides information on the transplantation and donation processes, living donations, support groups, transplant trends, living with a transplant, and much more.

NUTRITIONAL SUPPLEMENT PROVIDERS

BioInnovations
Phone: 888-442-6161
Website: www.bioinnovations.net

This company offers a range of nutritional supplements, including probiotics, natural anti-inflammatories, and other products.

Bio3 Research
1655 N. Main Street
Walnut Creek, CA 94545
Website: www.bio3research.com

A pharmaceutical company, Bio3 Research has developed a number of products for specific disorders, including Biocysan, a time-release form of cysteine designed to restore glutathione in people with Stage 5 kidney disease.

Kibow Biotech, Inc.
4629 West Chester Pike
Newtown Square, PA 19073
Phone: 610-353-5131
Website: www.kibowbiotech.com

Kibow produces Renadyl, a probiotic supplement that includes strains of microorganisms which have been shown to remove toxic waste products from the gastrointestinal tract.

LifeTime Vitamins

San Clemente, CA 92672

Phone: 800-333-6168

Website: www.lifetimevitamins.com

LifeTime offers a variety of supplements, including the protein powder Life's Basics Plant Protein, which provides antioxidant, anti-inflammatory, and muscle-building support.

Pure Formulas

11800 NW 102 Road, Suite 2

Medley, FL 33178

Phone: 800-383-6008

Website: www.pureformulas.com

Pure Formulas distributes a wide variety of supplements, including an excellent Life Extension product that combines glutathione, cysteine, and vitamin C.

$\mathcal{R}$eferences

Chapter 1

Alpert, M.A., Ravenscraft, M.D. "Pericardial involvement in end-stage renal disease." *Am J Med Sci*. Apr 2003; 325(4): 228–36.

Goovaerts, T., Jadoul, M., Goffin, E. "Influence of a pre-dialysis education programme (PDEP) on the mode of renal replacement therapy." *Nephrol Dial Transplant*. Sep 2005; 20(9): 1842–7.

Moss, A.H. "Ethical principles and processes guiding dialysis decision-making." *Clin Am Soc Nephrol*. Sep 2011; 6(9): 2313–7.

Ranganathan, N., Friedman, E.A., Tam, P., Rao, V., Ranganathan, P., Dheer, R. "Probiotic dietary supplementation in patients with stage 3 and 4 chronic kidney disease: a 6-month pilot scale trial in Canada." *Curr Med Res Opin*. Aug 2009; 25(8): 1919–30.

Shah, R.V., Givertz, M.M. "Managing acute renal failure in patients with acute decompensated heart failure: the cardiorenal syndrome." *Curr Heart Fail Rep*. Sep 2009; 6(3): 176–81.

Chapter 2

Boateng, E.A., East, L. "The impact of dialysis modality on quality of life: a systematic review." *J Ren Care*. Dec 2011; 37(4): 190–200.

Cheung, A.K., Sarnak, M.J., Yan, G., et al. "Cardiac diseases in maintenance hemodialysis patients: results of the HEMO Study." *Kidney Int*. Jun 2004; 65(6): 2380–9.

Doss, S., Schiller, B. "Dialysis overnight: in-center nocturnal hemodialysis programs showing growth." *Nephrol News Issues*. Jul 2011; 25(8): 22, 24, 26.

Hoenich, N.A., Ronco, C. "Perspectives in home hemodialysis therapy."*Contrib Nephrol.* 2011; 171: 25–9

Masterson, R. "The advantages and disadvantages of home hemodialysis." *Hemodial Int.* Jul 2008; 12 Suppl 1: S16–20.

Vilar, E., Farrington, K. "Emerging importance of residual renal function in end-stage renal failure." *Semin Dial.* Sep 2011; 24(5): 487–94.

Chapter 3

Allon, M., Litovsky, S., Young, C.J., et al. "Medial fibrosis, vascular calcification, intimal hyperplasia, and arteriovenous fistula maturation." *Am J Kidney Dis.* Sep 2011; 58(3): 437–43

Basel, H., Ekim, H., Odabasi, D., Kiymaz, A., Aydin, C., Dostbil, A. "Basilic vein transposition fistulas versus prosthetic bridge grafts in patients with end-stage renal failure." *Ann Vasc Surg.* Jul 2011; 25(5): 634–9.

Choy, K.J., Deng, Y.M., Hou, J.Y., et al. "Coenzyme Q(10) supplementation inhibits aortic lipid oxidation but fails to attenuate intimal thickening in balloon-injured New Zealand white rabbits." *Free Radic Biol Med.* Aug 2003; 35(3): 300–9.

Diskin, C.J. "The use of new concepts in vascular physiology and pharmacology to improve hemodialysis access outcomes." *Minerva Urol Nefrol.* Dec 2010; 62(4):387–410.

Ervo, S., Cavatorta, F., Zollo, A. "Implantation of permanent jugular catheters in patients on regular dialysis treatment: ten years' experience." *J Vasc Access.* Apr–June 2001; 2(2): 68–72.

Huang, B.F., Wang, W., Fu, Y.C., et al. "The effect of quercetin on neointima formation in a rat artery balloon injury model." 2009; 205(8): 515–23.

Lee, T., Barker, J., Allon, M. "Associations with predialysis vascular access management." *Am J Kidney Dis.* Jun 2004; 43(6): 1008–13.

Malik, G.H., Al-Harbi, A.S., Al-Mohaya, S.A., et al. "Chronic peritoneal dialysis a single-center experience." *Perit Dial Int.* Dec 2003; 23 Suppl 2: S188–91.

Rehman, R., Schmidt, R.J., Moss, A.H. "Ethical and legal obligation to avoid long-term tunneled catheter access." *Clin J Am Soc Nephrol.* Feb 2009; 4(2): 456–60.

Rosenblum, A., Mollicone, D., Wingard, R., Lacson, E., Jr. "Getting patients and renal staff to embrace 'fistula first/catheter last.' "*Nephrol News Issues.* Aug 2011; 25(9): 26–30.

Zou, J., Huang, Y., Cao, K., et al. "Effect of resveratrol on intimal hyperplasia after endothelial denudation in an experimental rabbit model." *Life Sci.* Dec 1, 2000; 68(2): 153–63.

Chapter 4

Anees, M.I., Ibrahim, M. "Anemia and hypoalbuminemia at initiation of hemodialysis as risk factor for survival of dialysis patients." *J Coll Physicians Surg Pak.* Dec 2009; 19(12): 776–80.

Bamgbola, O.F. "Pattern of resistance to erythropoietin-stimulating agents in chronic kidney disease." *Kidney Int.* Sep 2011; 80(5): 464–74.

Farag, Y.M., Keithi-Reddy, S.R., Mittal, B.V., et al. "Anemia, inflammation and health-related quality of life in chronic kidney disease patients." *Clin Nephrol.* June 2011; 75(6): 524–33.

Jean, G., Terrat, J.C., Vanel, T., et al. "Daily oral 25-hydroxycholecalciferol supplementation for vitamin D deficiency in haemodialysis patients: effects on mineral metabolism and bone markers." *Nephrol Dial Transplant.* Nov 2008; 23(11): 3670–6.

Kessler, E., Ritchey, N.P., Castro, F., et al. "Urea reduction ratio and urea kinetic modeling: a mathematical analysis of changing dialysis parameters." *Am J Nephrol.* 1998; 18(6): 471–7.

Kumar, V.A., Kujubu, D.A., Sim, J.J. "Vitamin D supplementation and recombinant human erythropoietin utilization in vitamin D-deficient hemodialysis patients." *J Nephrol.* Jan–Feb 2011; 24(1): 98–105.

Mohammed, I., Hutchison, A.J. "Oral phosphate binders for the management of serum phosphate levels in dialysis patients." *J Ren Care.* Mar 2009; 35 Suppl 1: 65–70.

Paganini, E.P. "Overview of anemia associated with chronic renal disease: primary and secondary mechanisms." *Semin Nephrol.* Mar 1989; 9(1 Suppl 1): 3–8.

Chapter 5

Frazão, J.M., Messa, P., Mellotte, G.J., et al. "Cinacalcet reduces plasma intact parathyroid hormone, serum phosphate and calcium levels in patients with secondary hyperparathyroidism irrespective of its severity." *Clin Nephrol.* Sep 2011; 76(3): 233–43.

Hosaka, K., Kazama, J.J., Yamamoto, S., et al. "Alterations in serum phosphate levels predict the long-term response to intravenous calcitriol therapy in dialysis patients with secondary hyperparathyroidism." *J Bone Miner Metab.* 2008; 26(2): 185–90

Loughnan, A., Ali, G.R., Abeygunasekara, S.C. "Comparison of the therapeutic efficacy of epoetin beta and epoetin alfa in maintenance phase hemodialysis patients." *Ren Fail.* 2011; 33(3): 373–5.

McMurray, J.J., Uno, H., Jarolim, P., et al. "Predictors of fatal and nonfatal cardiovascular events in patients with type 2 diabetes mellitus, chronic kidney disease, and anemia: an analysis of the Trial to Reduce cardiovascular Events with Aranesp (darbepoetin-alfa) Therapy (TREAT)." *Am Heart J.* Oct 2011; 162(4): 748–755.e3.

Chapter 6

Abol-Enein, H., Gheith, O.A., Barakat, N., et al. "Ionized alkaline water: new strategy for management of metabolic acidosis in experimental animals." *Ther Apher Dial*. Jun 2009; 13(3): 220–4.

Elming, M.B., Hornum, M., Feldt-Rasmussen, B., et al. "Cardiac autonomic neuropathy in patients with uraemia is not related to pre-diabetes." *Dan Med Bull*. Mar 2011; 58(3): A4244.

Ferrario, M., Moissl, U., Garzotto, F., et al. "Study of the autonomic response in hemodialysis patients with different fluid overload levels." *Conf Proc IEEE Eng Med Biol Soc*. 2010; 2010: 3796–9.

Mitchell, S. "Estimated dry weight (EDW): aiming for accuracy." *Nephrol Nurs J*. Oct 2002; 29(5): 421–8.

Raimann, J., Liu, L., Tyagi, S., et al. "A fresh look at dry weight." *Hemodial Int*. Oct 2008; 12(4): 395–405.

Sahni, V., Rosa, R.M., Batlle, D. "Potential benefits of alkali therapy to prevent GFR loss: time for a palatable 'solution' for the management of CKD." *Kidney Int*. Dec 2010; 78(11): 1065–7.

Wesson, D.E., Simoni, J. "Acid retention during kidney failure induces endothelin and aldosterone production which lead to progressive GFR decline, a situation ameliorated by alkali diet." *Kidney Int*. Dec 2010; 78(11): 1128–35

Chapter 7

Hörl, M.P., Hörl, W.H. "Drug therapy for hypertension in hemodialysis patients." *Semin Dial*. Jul–Aug 2004; 17(4): 288–94.

Kindler, J. "Torsemide in advanced renal failure." *Cardiovasc Drugs Ther*. Jan 1993; 7 Suppl 1: 75–80.

Snyder, R.W., Berns, J.S. "Use of insulin and oral hypoglycemic medications in patients with diabetes mellitus and advanced kidney disease." *Semin Dial*. Sep–Oct 2004; 17(5): 365–70.

Suzuki, H., Kanno, Y., Kaneko, K., et al. "Comparison of the effects of angiotensin receptor antagonist, angiotensin converting enzyme inhibitor, and their combination on regression of left ventricular hypertrophy of diabetes type 2 patients on recent onset hemodialysis therapy." *Ther Apher Dial*. Aug 2004; 8(4): 320–7.

Zheng, S., Nath, V., Coyne, D.W. "ACE inhibitor-based, directly observed therapy for hypertension in hemodialysis patients." *Am J Nephrol*. 2007; 27(5): 522–9.

Chapter 8

Bolland, M.J., Grey, A., Avenell, A., et al. "Calcium supplements with or without vitamin D and risk of cardiovascular events: reanalysis of the Women's Health Initiative limited access dataset and meta-analysis." *BMJ*. Apr 19, 2011; 342: d2040.

Castilla, P., Echarri, R., Dávalos, A., et al. "Concentrated red grape juice exerts antioxidant, hypolipidemic, and anti-inflammatory effects in both hemodialysis patients and healthy subjects." *Am J Clin Nutr.* Jul 2006; 84(1): 252–62.

Chang, J.W., Lee, E.K., Kim, T.H., et al. "Effects of alpha-lipoic acid on the plasma levels of asymmetric dimethylarginine in diabetic end-stage renal disease patients on hemodialysis: a pilot study." *Am J Nephrol.* 2007; 27(1): 70–4.

Debska-Slizień, A., Kawecka, A., Wojnarowski, K., et al. "Carnitine content in different muscles of patients receiving maintenance hemodialysis." *J Ren Nutr.* Jul 2007; 17(4): 275–81

Dhanasekaran, M., Ren, J. "The emerging role of coenzyme Q-10 in aging, neurodegeneration, cardiovascular disease, cancer and diabetes mellitus." *Curr Neurovasc Res.* Dec 2005; 2(5): 447–59.

Domański, M., Ciechanoski, K. "Sarcopenia: a major challenge in elderly patients with end-stage renal disease." *J Aging Res.* 2012; 2012: 754739.

Evans, A.M., Faull, R.J., Nation, R.L., et al. "Impact of hemodialysis on endogenous plasma and muscle carnitine levels in patients with end-stage renal disease." *Kidney Int.* Oct 2004; 66(4): 1527–34.

Fusaro, M., Crepaldi, G., Maggi, S., et al. "Vitamin K, bone fractures, and vascular calcifications in chronic kidney disease: an important but poorly studied relationship." *J Endocrinol Invest.* Apr 2011; 34(4): 317–23.

Handelman, G.J. "New insight on vitamin C in patients with chronic kidney disease." *J Ren Nutr.* Jan 2011; 21(1): 110–2.

Kalantar-Zadeh, K., Braglia, A., Chow, J., et al. "An anti-inflammatory and antioxidant nutritional supplement for hypoalbuminemic hemodialysis patients: a pilot/feasibility study." *J Ren Nutr.* Jul 2005; 15(3): 318–31.

Kristal, B., et al. "One year of pomegranate juice consumption decreases oxidative stress, inflammation, and infections in hemodialysis patients." *ASN 2010: Abstract TH-FC059.*

McDonnell, M.G., Archbold, G.P. "Plasma ubiquinol/cholesterol ratios in patients with hyperlipidaemia, those with diabetes mellitus and in patients requiring dialysis." *Clin Chim Acta.* Sep 30, 1996; 253(1–2): 117–26.

Movilli, E., Viola, B.F., Camerini, C., Mazzola, G., et al. "Correction of metabolic acidosis on serum albumin and protein catabolism in hemodialysis patients." *J Ren Nutr.* Mar 2009; 19(2): 172–7.

Nakashima, A., Yorioka, N., Doi, S., et al. "Effects of vitamin K2 in hemodialysis patients with low serum parathyroid hormone levels." *Bone.* Mar 2004; 34(3): 579–83.

Nguyen-Khoa, T., Massy, Z.A., De Bandt, J.P., et al. "Oxidative stress and haemodialysis: role of inflammation and duration of dialysis treatment." *Nephrol Dial Transplant.* Feb 2001; 16(2): 335–40.

Omran, H., McCarter, D., St Cyr, J., et al. "D-ribose aids congestive heart failure patients." *Exp Clin Cardiol.* Summer 2004; 9(2): 117–8.

Richter, A., Kuhlmann, M.K., Seibert, E., et al. "Vitamin C deficiency and secondary hyperparathyroidism in chronic haemodialysis patients." *Nephrol Dial Transplant.* Jun 2008; 23(6): 2058–63.

Sakurabayashi, T., Miyazaki, S., Yuasa, Y., et al. "L-carnitine supplementation decreases the left ventricular mass in patients undergoing hemodialysis." *Circ J.* Jun 2008; 72(6): 926–31.

Schlieper, G., Westenfeld, R., Krüger, T., et al. "Circulating nonphosphorylated carboxylated matrix gla protein predicts survival in ESRD." *J Am Soc Nephrol.* Feb 2011; 22(2): 387–95.

Sharma, A., Gadepally, P. "Nutritional therapy to attenuate inflammation in HD patients: fact or fiction?" *Nephrol News Issues.* Jan 2010; 24(1): 26–9.

Shin, J.I., Park, S.J., Kim, J.H. "Could intradialytic hypotension be due to low baseline magnesium levels or inflammation in hemodialysis patients?" *Hemodial Int.* Apr 2011; 15(2): 301–2

Sundell, M.B., Cavanaugh, K.L., Wu, P., et al. "Oral protein supplementation alone improves anabolism in a dose-dependent manner in chronic hemodialysis patients." *J Ren Nutri.* Sep 2009; 19(5): 412—21.

Usberti, M., Lima, G., Arisi, M., et al. "Effect of exogenous reduced glutathione on the survival of red blood cells in hemodialyzed patients." *J Nephrol.* Sep–Oct 1997; 10(5): 261–5.

Ziegler, D., Low, P.A., Litchy, W.J., et al. "Efficacy and safety of antioxidant treatment with α-lipoic acid over 4 years in diabetic polyneuropathy: the NATHAN 1 trial." *Diabetes Care.* Sep 2011; 34(9): 2054–60.

Zou, J., Huang, Y., Cao, K., et al. "Effect of resveratrol on intimal hyperplasia after endothelial denudation in an experimental rabbit model." *Life Sciences.* Dec 1, 2000; 68(2): 153–63.

Chapter 9

Bronich, L., Te, T., Shetye, K., et al. "Successful treatment of hypoalbuminemic hemodialysis patients with a modified regimen of oral essential amino acids." *J Ren Nutr.* Oct 2001; 11(4): 194–201.

Brookhyser-Hogan, J. *The Vegetarian Diet for Kidney Disease: Preserving Kidney Function with Plant-Based Eating.* Laguna Beach, CA: Basic Health Publications, 2010.

Domański, M., Ciechanowski, K. "Sarcopenia: a major challenge in elderly patients with end-stage renal disease." *J Aging Res.* 2012; 2012: 754739.

Kalantar-Zadeh, K., Braglia, A., Chow, J., et al. "An anti-inflammatory and antioxidant nutritional supplement for hypoalbuminemic hemodialysis patients: a pilot/feasibility study." *J Ren Nutr.* Jul 2005; 15(3): 318–31.

Movilli, E., Viola, B.F., Camerini, C., Mazzola, G., et al. "Correction of metabolic acidosis on serum albumin and protein catabolism in hemodialysis patients." *J Ren Nutr.* Mar 2009; 19(2): 172–7.

Sharma, A., Gadepally, P. "Nutritional therapy to attenuate inflammation in HD patients: fact or fiction?" *Nephrol News Issues.* Jan 2010; 24(1): 26–9.

Sherman, RA. "Dietary phosphate restriction and protein intake in dialysis patients: a misdirected focus." *Semin Dial.* Jan–Feb 2007; 20(1): 16–8.

Sundell, M.B., Cavanaugh, K.L., Wu, P., et al. "Oral protein supplementation alone improves anabolism in a dose-dependent manner in chronic hemodialysis patients." *J Ren Nutri.* Sep 2009; 19(5): 412—21.

Westra, W.M., Kopple, J.D., Krediet, R.T., et al. "Dietary protein requirements and dialysate protein losses in chronic peritoneal dialysis patients." *Perit Dial Int.* Mar–Apr 2007; 27(2): 192–5.

Chapter 10

Bossola, M., Vulpio, C., Tazza, L. "Fatigue in chronic dialysis patients." *Semin Dial.* Sep 2011; 24(5): 550–5.

Bullani, R., El-Housseini, Y., Giordano, F., et al. "Effect of intradialytic resistance band exercise on physical function in patients on maintenance hemodialysis: a pilot study." *J Ren Nutr.* Jan 2011; 21(1): 61–5.

Dijoseph, J., Cavendish, R. "Expanding the dialogue on prayer relevant to holistic care." *Holist Nurs Pract.* Jul–Aug 2005; 19(4): 147–54.

Ikizler, T.A. "Exercise as an anabolic intervention in patients with end-stage renal disease." *J Ren Nutr.* Jan 2011; 21(1): 52–6.

Mattison, D. "The forgotten spirit: integration of spirituality in health care." *Nephrol News Issues.* Feb 2006; 20(2): 30–2.

Tentori, F., Elder, S.J., Thumma, J., et al. "Physical exercise among participants in the Dialysis Outcomes and Practice Patterns Study (DOPPS): correlates and associated outcomes." *Nephrol Dial Transplant.* Sep 2010; 25(9): 3050–62.

Chapter 11

Knoll, G. "Trends in kidney transplantation over the past decade." *Drugs.* 2008; 68 Suppl 1: 3–10.

O'Connor, K.J., Delmonico, F.L. "Increasing the supply of kidneys for transplantation." *Semin Dial.* Nov–Dec 2005; 18(6): 460–2.

Veroux, M., Corona, D., Veroux, P. "Kidney transplantation: future challenges." *Minerva Chir.* Feb 2009; 64(1): 75–100.

Index

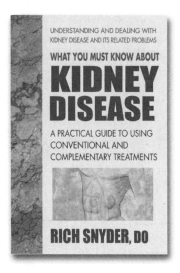

WHAT YOU MUST KNOW ABOUT KIDNEY DISEASE

A Practical Guide to Using Conventional and Complementary Treatments

Rich Snyder, DO

While the news that you or someone you love has kidney disease can be shocking, for over 26 million Americans, it is a reality. After the initial diagnosis, patients and families usually have a myriad of questions about treatment options. *What You Must Know About Kidney Disease* is designed not only to answer all your questions, but also to provide the up-to-date information you need to evaluate and choose both conventional treatments and complementary therapies.

The book is divided into three parts. Part One provides an overview of the kidneys' structure and function and discusses common kidney disorders. It also guides you in asking your doctor questions that will help you better understand both the status of your health and your prognosis. Part Two examines kidney problems and their conventional treatments. Part Three presents an in-depth look at the most effective complementary therapies available, from simple lifestyle changes to acupuncture, nutritional and herbal supplementation, osteopathic manipulation, and more.

There is so much you can do to positively affect both your kidney health and your overall well-being. *What You Must Know About Kidney Disease* provides you with the knowledge you need to be a wise participant in your own health care.

$17.95 • 192 pages • 6 x 9-inch quality paperback • ISBN 978-0-7570-0326-4

THE ACID-ALKALINE FOOD GUIDE

A Quick Reference to Foods & Their Effect on pH Levels

Susan E. Brown, PhD, CCN,
and Larry Trivieri, Jr.

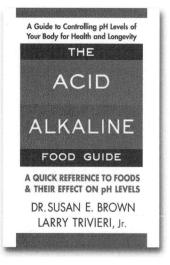

In the last few years, researchers around the world have reported the importance of acid-alkaline balance. When the body enjoys pH balance, you experience radiant good health. When the body is not in balance, the disease process begins, resulting in problems ranging from bone loss to premature aging and more. The key to a healthy pH is proper diet, but for a long time, acid-alkaline food guides have included only a small number of foods. Or they did, until now.

The Acid-Alkaline Food Guide is a complete resource for people who want to widen their food choices. The book begins by explaining how the acid-alkaline environment of the body is influenced by foods. It then presents a list of thousands of foods and their acid-alkaline effects. Included are not only single foods, such as fruits and vegetables, but also popular combination and even fast foods, like burgers and fries. In each case, you'll not only discover whether a food is acidifying or alkalizing, but you'll learn the *degree* to which that food affects the body. Informative insets guide you in choosing the food that's right for you.

The first book of its kind, *The Acid-Alkaline Food Guide* will quickly become the resource you turn to at home, in restaurants, and whenever you want to select a food that can help you reach your health and dietary goals.

$7.95 • 208 pages • 4 x 7-inch mass paperback • ISBN 978-0-7570-0280-9

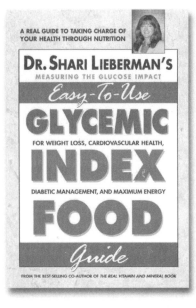

A REAL GUIDE TO TAKING CHARGE OF YOUR HEALTH THROUGH NUTRITION

DR. SHARI LIEBERMAN'S

MEASURING THE GLUCOSE IMPACT

Easy-To-Use

GLYCEMIC

FOR WEIGHT LOSS, CARDIOVASCULAR HEALTH,

INDEX

DIABETIC MANAGEMENT, AND MAXIMUM ENERGY

FOOD

Guide

FROM THE BEST-SELLING CO-AUTHOR OF *THE REAL VITAMIN AND MINERAL BOOK*

GLYCEMIC INDEX FOOD GUIDE

For Weight Loss, Cardiovascular Health, Diabetic Management, and Maximum Energy

Dr. Shari Lieberman

The glycemic index (GI) is an important nutritional tool. By indicating how quickly a given food triggers a rise in blood sugar, the GI enables you to choose foods that can help you manage a variety of conditions and improve your overall health.

Written by leading nutritionist Dr. Shari Lieberman, this book was designed as an easy-to-use guide to the glycemic index. The book first answers commonly asked questions, ensuring that you truly understand the GI and know how to use it. It then provides both the glycemic index and the glycemic load of hundreds of foods and beverages, including raw foods, cooked foods, and many combination and prepared foods. Whether you are interested in controlling your glucose levels to manage your diabetes, lose weight, increase your heart health, or simply enhance your well-being, the *Glycemic Index Food Guide* is the best place to start.

$7.95 • 160 pages • 4 x 7-inch mass paperback • ISBN 978-0-7570-0245-8